Keto Diet

Table of Contents

Introduction

The Keto Diet is the new trend in smart eating to lose weight – the reason why it has been able to capture such attention is because of its unique approach. The Keto Diet is all about eating high contents of fat and low contents of carb. When people first hear this they're always surprised because how can eating more fat make us slimmer? Well, that's because fats have been heavily stigmatized which is why all of us believe that it's only fats that make us fat when actually it's the carbs and sugars that we consume every day.

There are fats that are terrible for your body and you should avoid them, but there are also some good fats that help your body to absorb more vitamins and minerals from the food you consume. A high-fat diet doesn't just help you to lose weight, but also improves your cognitive abilities, cholesterol and even provides safety against many diseases.

The purpose of a keto is to make your eating habits a little more natural so that you stop consuming food that is artificial and fattening and instead consume food that is full of fats such as butter, cheese, nuts and fish.

In this book, you will learn everything about the keto diet – what it is all about, how it works, what are the benefits, how to follow it and how to keep yourself motivated.

Thanks again for purchasing this book, I hope you enjoy it!

Chapter One:
Ketogenic Diet Basics

Ketogenic diet is a diet that places and trains your body to be in a state wherein it primarily uses fat for energy. It achieves this through a natural metabolic process of your body called Ketosis that uses fat to create fuel for your body. A ketogenic diet has many similarities to the Atkins diet and many other low-carb diets. It has been known by several different names like low carb high fat, low carb diet and of course, the ketogenic diet.

The ketogenic diet can be implemented by discarding most of the sugars and starches in your diet and by eating healthy fats, moderate amounts of protein and very low carbs. With little carbohydrates in your diet, your body does not receive enough glucose to keep up with your body's caloric requirements. This eventually results in decreasing blood sugar levels in your body as it uses up glucose for its functions. When you eat foods that are high in carbs, your body automatically produces insulin and glucose. Insulin is made to process the glucose that is in your bloodstream by moving it around the body. Glucose is easy for your body to convert and be used for energy. Therefore, it gets chosen over all other energy sources.

As blood sugar level decreases, it looks for the stored glycogen present in your body and breaks it down to glucose and dissolves it in your blood to be distributed throughout your body. However, glycogen stores would also eventually run out. And when it does, your body would start to use fats as a source of energy for functions in its different parts and produce ketones when the liver processes it. Since glucose is used as the primary energy source, the fat in your body isn't needed and gets stored. With a normal, high carb diet, your body uses glucose as its main form of energy. By lowering the carb intake, the body is put into ketosis. These fats could come from the food that you eat, from your meals or from the fat that your body stores. This is what is called ketosis.

When you hit ketosis, your body starts being very efficient at burning fat to create energy. It turns fat in the liver into ketones that supply energy to the brain. Many studies have shown that a keto diet can help you to improve your health and lose some weight. It can also help with Alzheimer's disease, epilepsy, cancer and diabetes.

The primary advantage of following a ketogenic diet is that it restores the capability of your body to use both fat and glucose as fuel to meet its energy or caloric needs. Your body is designed to use both glucose and fat as fuel. However, due to eating a high carbohydrate diet for most of their lives, many people lack the ability to use fat for the body's energy needs. This results in bodies that have a hard time maintaining a healthy weight and a healthy body fat percentage, both of which contribute to poor health. In fact, even if you are not overweight or obese, you may still have excess visceral fat, which is wrapped around your organs like your liver, pancreas and kidneys.

With a ketogenic diet, your body restores its flexibility to use both glucose and fat as fuel for its energy needs. This flexibility keeps your fat cells, both visceral and subcutaneous (the fat located under your skin and on top of your muscles), in check by using the stored energy found in those fat cells. This would, in turn, reduce the risks of having diseases involved with having high-fat stores, specifically visceral fat:

- Type 2 Diabetes
- Coronary Artery/ Heart Disease

- Colorectal Cancer
- Breast Cancer
- High Cholesterol
- High Blood Pressure
- Metabolic Syndrome
- Alzheimer's Disease
- Stroke
- Dementia

Other than decreasing risks of said diseases, this flexibility contributes to losing excess fat and weight in a manageable manner. Normally, while and after losing some weight, your body would feel less sated after eating the same meal you ate before the weight loss process started.

And in addition to this, you might feel an increase in appetite to compensate especially if you've been depriving yourself. However, when your body is in a state of ketosis, ketones help your body manage the hormones that decrease your satiety after meals and increase your appetite and hunger. With this, you lose weight without fighting your body to gain it back through its natural responses as to what it believes to be starvation.

Moreover, being able to utilize glucose and fat for energy prevents you from experiencing the big swings that affect your mental focus, making you hungry and irritable. When glucose runs out, ketones are readily available to fuel your brain. Even better, ketones give your brain a boost, enabling you to have better focus and concentration.

Lastly, the ketogenic diet has long been used for therapy of epilepsy. This diet has been recommended for children with uncontrolled epilepsy since the 1920's. It only disappeared from popular practice when the anti-seizure medication was made available. However, unlike the anti-seizure medicine currently available, the ketogenic diet does not cause extreme side effects on patients; like drowsiness, reduced concentration, personality changes and reduced brain function.

Starting Information & Tips

The Standard Ketogenic Diet (SKD) means that 70 percent of your diet should be in the form of healthy fats, 25 percent in the form of protein and 5 percent of carbohydrates. The percentages would be based on your daily caloric requirement that is unique for every person. Since you may need to increase your caloric intake due to higher needs, you may increase the percentage of healthy fats in your diet and your body can still achieve ketosis.

Other variations of the ketogenic diet that are tweaked based on certain needs are listed down below:

Targeted Ketogenic Diet (TKD)

This type of ketogenic diet is recommended for those who engage in physical fitness. In TKD, 30 to 60 minutes before exercise, you would eat the entirety of your carbohydrates for the day in one meal. The idea of this approach is to use the energy provided in this carbohydrate meal for your fitness activities before it disrupts your body's state of ketosis.

Cyclic Ketogenic Diet (CKD)

This approach is intended for people who have a high rate of physical activities like athletes and bodybuilders. When following CKD, you switch between a ketogenic diet, and after that you follow it with a few days of high carbohydrate consumption (9 to 12 times the carbohydrates in SKD), more commonly called, "carb loading." This approach takes advantage of the body's response to high blood sugar levels from a high carbohydrate diet, which is to store it in the body's muscles and fat cells. Having this abundance of stored energy and the body able to utilize both glucose and fat for energy, it can use this energy to keep the body going during high rates of physical activity.

High-Protein Ketogenic Diet

This is a method used to ease into a Standard Ketogenic Diet when the weight is beyond the normal levels. In this approach, your protein consumption in an SKD is increased by 10 percent and your fat consumption is reduced by 10 percent. This helps those with obesity to help suppress their appetite and reduce their food intake.

Restricted Ketogenic Diet:

This method was successfully used for a brain tumor patient. In this approach, carbohydrate and calorie intake are restricted for your body to deplete glycogen stores and to start producing ketones. Since cancer cells can only feed on glucose, they are starved to death while your body thrives on ketones. It starts with a water fasting regimen and proceeds to only have a Ketogenic Diet of 600 calories a day. After two months, ketosis is in full effect and no discernable brain tumor tissue can be detected.

Only the high protein ketogenic and the standard diets have had extensive studies done on them. The targeted and cyclical diets are more advanced and are only used by athletes and bodybuilders. Even though there are several different types of this diet, the standard ketogenic diet has been researched the most and is, therefore, the one that is usually recommended.

The reason why ketogenic diets are effective lies in the functional property of fat adaption. Your body needs to be told that it has to derive its energy from fats. The biggest challenge in this regard is to keep the body programmed to this state, on a regular basis. In order to maintain ketosis, here are a few tips that you must pay heed to.

Tip 1: Drink Enough Water

You must drink a healthy amount of water to maintain a healthy body. This is a fact that all of us know and are told about time and again. However, it has also proven to be the most difficult advice to follow. The modern lifestyle is so consuming that we mostly forget simple things like keeping our bodies hydrated and eating our meals on time. It is a good idea to drink around 4 glasses of water, first thing in the morning and another 4 glasses of water before the clock strikes noon.

Tip 2: Fast Once In A While

Like we said, our bodies fail to use up the fat stores because we never, ever fast. The body is pre-programmed to run ketosis as and when the body starves. Therefore, if you are finding it hard to get your body into ketosis or maintain the ketosis state of the body, you can fast intermittently. Fasting also helps in reducing food intake and manages appetites and cravings, both of which are crucial for your diet plan. However, be sure to go on a low-carb diet for a few days before fasting intermittently. The sudden lack of sugar in the body may land you up in a hypoglycemic state.

A daylong fast can be easily broken down into two phases. The first phase extends from the first meal you consume to the last meal you eat for the day. This is the build-up phase. The second phase, which extends from your last meal for the day to the first meal of the next day, is the cleansing phase. Ideally, the cleansing phase must be longer than the build-up phase. Whenever you fast, be sure to keep your body hydrated and eat good fats like butter and coconut oil. These additions play an instrumental role in boosting up the ketone production of the body and help to maintain a healthy insulin level.

Tip 3: Add Good Salts

The high insulin levels of the body, when it is in glycolysis, affect the functioning of the kidney in such a manner that the body retains sodium. As a result, the sodium-potassium ratio destabilizes. This is why most people are advised to reduce their sodium intake. On the other hand, when on a ketogenic diet, the insulin levels are normal and the kidney functioning allows sodium excretion more effectively.

As a result, the body needs sodium to ensure proper functioning. Never make the mistake of avoiding salts when running your body on a ketogenic diet. There are several ways by which you can increase the sodium levels of the body. Some of the best ways include having broth, eating sprouted pumpkin seeds, eating cucumber as part of the salad for natural sodium and adding a pinch of salt to almost everything you eat.

Tip 4: Exercise

Regular exercise can play a crucial role in maintaining the ketosis state of the body and avoiding deposition of glucose in body parts. Exercise allows activation of glucose transport molecules that facilitate deposition of glucose in the muscles and liver. Exercises like the ones used for resistance training also facilitate the maintenance of normal blood sugar levels.

It is important to understand in this context that overdoing exercise can result in the release of stress hormones. This, in turn, increases sugar levels of the body and destabilizes the ketosis state of the body. Regular and 'just-enough' exercise can be a great way to keep you on track.

Tip 5: Avoid Too Much Protein

Most regular diet programs recommend higher protein intake. However, excessive protein intake can initiate what is called gluconeogenesis, which again generates glucose. If you feel that your body is no longer able to maintain the ketosis state, you must take a keen look at the number of proteins that you are consuming. You may have more success with a much lower protein intake.

Tip 6: Choose What You Eat Wisely

Although the ketogenic diet recommends a reduced carbohydrate intake, it is not a good idea to remove carbs from the diet completely. Therefore, the inclusion of starchy vegetables and citric fruit is a good idea. On an odd day when you are off-ketosis, you can consume berries and potatoes. However, when on ketosis, be sure to avoid sweet potato and berry-type fruit completely.

Tip 7: Reduce Stress

Stress is the root cause of most of the problems that your body's face. In fact, an increase in the stress hormones in the body can pull you off ketosis because it increases the sugar levels substantially. Therefore, maintaining a ketosis state can be an uphill task if you are going through stressful times in your life. Managing stress is an important facet of the ketogenic diet. Adopt strategies that keep your stress levels in check if you wish to make your ketogenic diet work. In line with this objective, having adequate amounts of daily sleep and maintaining a stable lifestyle is also essential.

Who should follow this diet?

The keto diet is known in popular discourse only for weight loss, but it's about much more. In this section, we will look at who should follow this diet -

Epileptic Patients

The ketogenic diet was originally developed in the early 1900s as a means of controlling seizures in children. Fasting was long a treatment in treating epilepsy and doctors found that a high-fat diet helped mimic the metabolic response of fasting. They began treating epileptic children by feeding them a diet in which up to 90% of the calories came from fat and found a marked reduction in the seizures. Half of the children fed a ketogenic diet had a reduced number of seizures and about one in seven had a complete elimination of seizures altogether.

Some studies suggest that the ketones created by the ketogenic diet are the reason it is successful in treating epilepsy. Others believe that the depletion of glucose is the reason for its success. Whatever the reason, it has proven to be effective when medication has not.

The ketogenic diet, especially when used to treat seizures, is very intense and highly controlled and can be difficult for children to follow. Doctors usually only recommend it after multiple rounds of medication have proven unsuccessful. However, many of the epileptic children who are put on the ketogenic diet for two years or longer experience a reduction or elimination of seizures, even after they cease eating it. It does not seem to have the same effect in treating epileptic teenagers and adults, possibly because it is so strict and difficult to follow. However, they can still be treated with it as long as they are willing to follow it exactly.

The ketogenic diet for epilepsy is stricter than the ketogenic diet that many people are adhering to boost their health. Rather than a 70% fat this one

11

requires 90% fats. Side effects can include stunted growth, constipation, kidney stones, weight loss and weaker bones. If the side effects become too much, a less intense but possibly less-effective diet, such as modified Atkins, can be implemented instead.

When an epileptic patient is starting out on the ketogenic diet, he or she may need to spend a few days in the hospital for monitoring to see what effects the diet is having. Close medical monitoring will be required, including keeping a food diary, corresponding with a dietitian and getting tested every one to three months. Hyper-vigilance for carbs is required, as they can show up in some very unexpected places. For example, most kinds of toothpaste and mouthwashes contain carbs.

Parents who place their epileptic children on a ketogenic diet will have to make substantial lifestyle changes. They will have to be able to implement the diet in such a way that the epileptic child does not see it as "unfair". He or she may see siblings enjoying sweets and feel left out. All caregivers, including babysitters, teachers and other family members, will have to be aware of the strict diet. Relatives who may want to "spoil" the child by giving him or her treats at family reunions will have to understand how serious the diet is, as one simple misstep or "cheat" can trigger seizures. Some creative ideas for handling these difficult situations include using treats other than food, such as toys, fun outings, or television time. Before Halloween one year, one dad of an epileptic child on the ketogenic diet sent out a letter to all of the homes in his neighborhood that explained why his son couldn't have candy and included a toy to give him instead. The heartwarming letter went viral.

When a medical professional advises getting off the ketogenic diet in favor of a more traditional diet that includes more carbs and protein, the transition will need to be made gradually. Especially in children, the body has become so adjusted to the ketogenic diet that the metabolic changes can be difficult to adapt to.

Type 1 Diabetics

Unlike Type 2 diabetes, Type 1 diabetes is actually an autoimmune disease in which the immune system attacks the pancreas and destroys the beta cells that detect blood sugar and create insulin. As a result, the body's cells are unable to absorb any glucose and blood sugar can build up to dangerously high levels. Type 1 diabetics usually must administer insulin through injections and constantly monitor their blood sugar levels to make sure they are within a safe range. While many people are diagnosed with it as children, half of those diagnosed are over the age of 30.

There are many complications that people with Type 1 diabetes can experience, possibly as a result of the autoimmune dysfunction rather than insulin deficiency. High blood pressure and blood sugar levels can lead to eye damage, such as diabetic retinopathy, nerve damage, kidney damage and heart disease. The challenge in successfully responding to Type 1 diabetes is not only regulating blood sugar and insulin levels but also dealing with the autoimmune problems that can lead to further complications.

Lifestyle is the most important factor in managing Type 1 diabetes. Avoiding sugar, getting regular exercise, being
consistent with insulin injections and being aware of the symptoms of impending problems are some of the most crucial things. Lowering blood sugar, thereby lowering the need for insulin, can be very effective at managing the disease.
The ketogenic diet can be a powerful way of lowering blood sugar in patients with Type 1 diabetes. Many find that they are able to reduce their need for insulin by up to 80% or more.

When following a ketogenic diet with Type 1 diabetes, the person must be absolutely all in. There are no cheats allowed, as just one cheat meal can put the body in a dangerous, potentially deadly state known as ketoacidosis. This occurs when ketones build up in the blood, causing it to become more acidic.

The ketones, which are naturally present on the ketogenic diet, can build up to dangerously high levels as they react with the blood sugar. Diabetics on the ketogenic diet should closely monitor their ketone and glucose levels and remain carefully under a doctor's supervision.

Type 1 diabetics may need to follow a modified version of the ketogenic diet, which is more strictly controlled but more suited to the disease.

Type 2 Diabetics

Type 2 diabetes, also known as adult diabetes, is oftentimes the result of lifestyle choices that lead to chronically high levels of blood sugar, thereby leading to insulin resistance. While Type 1 diabetes is caused by the inability of the body to create insulin, Type 2 diabetes is the result of it being unable to use insulin. Increasingly unhealthy lifestyle choices are leading to children being diagnosed with Type 2 diabetes, whereby it was previously unheard of in people under the age of 50.

Diet, exercise and close monitoring of insulin levels are key to managing Type 2 diabetes. Complete lifestyle overhauls have led some people to completely reverse the symptoms and no longer need medication. The most obvious benefit is that the lowered blood sugar leads to less dependence on insulin.

The conundrum created by applying the ketogenic diet to Type 2 diabetes is that because so many people with the disease are overweight or obese, adopting a high-fat diet seems to be counterintuitive. After all, fat is a much more concentrated source of calories than carbs or protein, so it should actually lead to weight gain and exacerbate the person's health problems. However, that is a myth based on a misunderstanding of calories and the complex chemistry involved in metabolism. The fact is that not all calories are created equal and healthy fats, as opposed to carbs, can actually decrease your appetite so that you end up consuming fewer calories. Additionally, the decreased production of ghrelin, the hunger hormone and the increased production of leptin and amylin, the satiety hormones, generated by the state of ketosis further restrict the calorie intake.

As with Type 1 diabetes, people with Type 2 diabetes are at risk of developing ketoacidosis, so constant monitoring of blood sugar and ketones is important. Additionally, the ketogenic diet should be followed under a doctor's supervision.

Early-Stage Alzheimer's Patients

One of the biggest health concerns today is the risk of developing Alzheimer's disease. Alzheimer's seems to have a bit of a genetic component and is also linked with lifestyle factors. As previously mentioned, some researchers have come to call it Type 3 Diabetes because of its connection with insulin resistance and a buildup of glucose in the brain.

Preliminary studies, both in animal and human trials, indicate that the ketogenic diet is effective at restoring normal brain metabolism in people with early-stage Alzheimer's disease. It reduces and can even eliminate the buildup of unabsorbed glucose that leads to cell death while providing the brain with the superior energy provided by ketones. Ketones are able to provide all of the nutrients necessary for optimal brain function. At optimal levels they do not build up in the bloodstream, leading to the creation of the dangerous plaques and tangles that cause neurodegeneration.

As yet, there is no indication that the ketogenic diet can reverse Alzheimer's disease once it has begun. However, results so far are promising. Research over the past few decades has revealed that the brain has a high level of plasticity, meaning that neurons are able to regenerate, grow and adapt to changing needs. Ketones may be able to tap into this plasticity to help halt Alzheimer's in its tracks and future research into treatment for Alzheimer's will focus heavily on ketones.

People who are diagnosed with Alzheimer's disease tend to be older, usually over the age of 60, so implementing the changes required by the ketogenic diet can be difficult. Additionally, maintaining the person's lifestyle as much as possible is seen as a cornerstone in caring for someone with Alzheimer's, as consistency and normalcy can help deal with the emotional challenges that people with the disease face. Getting Alzheimer's patients to establish a ketogenic diet can be very difficult and will require the complete commitment of all caregivers.

People, who are at risk of developing Alzheimer's disease, because of preexisting insulin resistance, genetic factors, or environmental factors, may benefit from the ketogenic diet. It may prevent the brain decay that is characteristic of the disease.

Parkinson's Patients

Parkinson's disease is a neurodegenerative disorder caused by abnormal levels of the hormone dopamine. The dopamine-creating neurons die and the loss of dopamine results in the characteristic tremors that people with

Parkinson's experience. Additionally, they deal with problems such as depression, lack of clarity, forgetfulness and loss of physical function. The disease is progressive, so it gets worse over time. Medications are available to help manage the symptoms, but there is no cure.

Dysfunction in the mitochondria is believed to be a cause of the death of the dopamine-creating neurons, which leads to Parkinson's. The previous chapter already discussed the role of ketones in protecting and enhancing the mitochondria, so from this perspective, ketones may play a role in helping to treat Parkinson's patients. Preliminary studies in animals have shown that the ketogenic diet can improve mitochondrial function. In humans, a preliminary study has shown that one month on the ketogenic diet leads to decreased tremors, elevated mood, improved gait and increased energy.

People who are diagnosed with Parkinson's disease tend to be older, so implementing the intense lifestyle changes required by the ketogenic diet can be quite difficult. Those who participated in the preliminary testing had trouble staying on it and several quit, despite the potential for treatment. A gradual transition to the ketogenic diet may be helpful in maintaining it.

Cancer Patients

In addition to finding new medications that can potentially help cancer patients, much cancer research is now looking into the effects of diet and lifestyle as supplements to traditional treatments. Vegetable juicing and eating an organic-only diet has helped many cancer patients recover. New research is focusing on the potential of a ketogenic diet in helping to cure cancer.

One way that a ketogenic diet may benefit cancer patients is that sugar is all but eliminated. Sugar is basically what cancer cells thrive on; there is a direct correlation between sugar consumption and growth of tumors. By switching the body's energy source from glucose to ketones, the tumors become starved and may shrink.

Additionally, the benefits for mitochondrial metabolism may improve the responses of healthy cells and generate apoptosis, the body's method of intentionally destroying cancerous cells. Studies are showing that a ketogenic diet increases the oxidative stress on the mitochondria in cancer cells, making them more sensitive to chemotherapy and other traditional treatments.

Meanwhile, the mitochondria of the healthy cells are enhanced, making them less prone to the harmful effects of treatments. Cancer patients who want to adopt a ketogenic diet should consult with an oncologist who specializes in how a ketogenic diet can help with that particular type of cancer.

PCOS Patients

Polycystic ovarian syndrome, or PCOS, is a metabolic dysfunction that is closely correlated with insulin resistance. It leads to problems such as infertility, acne, dysmenorrhea (heavy periods that have intense cramping), amenorrhea (lack of periods) and hirsutism (irregular hair growth across the body). While the ovaries usually release an egg every 28 days, in women with PCOS, the eggs remain in the ovaries and turn into cysts. Over time, the cysts build up in both ovaries until there are dozens or even hundreds. Many women with PCOS treat their symptoms with medication, but the disease can also be managed and sometimes even reversed through diet.

Consistently high levels of blood sugar cause insulin resistance. The first step to treating PCOS through diet is by eliminating sugar, then reducing and eliminating all other carbs, as well. PCOS is also strongly correlated with obesity; some women develop PCOS and become obese because of the intense hormonal disruptions, while some obese women are more prone to developing PCOS. Another step towards treating the disease with diet is to lose weight. Because the weight gain tends to be at least partly hormonal, balancing the hormones is crucial.

The ketogenic diet can help women with PCOS to both balance their hormones and lose weight. Although clinical studies are few and small, case studies and anecdotal evidence regarding the success of low-carb diets in treating PCOS are impressive; the lowered insulin levels help to reverse insulin resistance and stabilize other hormone imbalances. It is not uncommon for women with PCOS who are on a low-carb diet to lose weight, achieve normal periods and even regain their fertility.

While there is little research as to the ketogenic diet specifically with women who have PCOS, preliminary results are promising. There are several foods on the ketogenic diet, such as fatty fish and nuts that are particularly helpful for those with the disease. If you have PCOS and want to try the ketogenic diet to see if it can help relieve your symptoms and even reverse the disease, talk with your endocrinologist about how it may benefit you.

People with Autism

Autism is a neurological disorder that has been on the rise, particularly in the United States. Its characteristic feature is impaired social interaction and cognitive development, including language development. The increased prevalence of autistic diagnoses has led many parents to be concerned about possible causes of autism. Some have even shunned life-saving vaccines because they are concerned that they may cause autism. Its causes seem to be varied and include genetic and environmental factors.

Treatment usually focuses on managing behavior with intense therapy; there is no known cure for autism. It is a lifelong condition and many adults with autism must either be cared for full time by a family member or live in a care home. The success of the ketogenic diet in treating neurological disorders has led to speculation about whether it may be able to benefit people with autism. Many diets have been applied to clinical studies for children with autism spectrum disorders, but the benefits seem to be minimal. However, the ketogenic diet seems to hold great promise and has already proven to help autistic children in some clinical trials.

It is not uncommon for people with autism to also suffer from seizures. The benefits of the ketogenic diet in treating seizures were described in the first section; someone with autism who also has seizures may experience diminished epileptic activity as a result of the ketogenic diet.

Autism spectrum disorders tend to display certain behaviors, including repetitive behaviors known as stimming and agitation. Mice with characteristics that mimic autism, such as repetitive behaviors and lack of social interaction, who were fed a ketogenic diet experienced reversals of the symptoms and behaved like normal mice. In clinical trials, autistic children fed a ketogenic diet experienced marked improvement in these behaviors and even showed an increase in social activity.

Autism also tends to have an effect on cognition. While some forms of autism, such as Asperger's syndrome, can lead to increased mental acuity, there is oftentimes a lack of executive function, which inhibits the person's ability to make connections between ideas. The ketogenic diet has been shown to help people with autism improve their cognitive process. This may be because it promotes the neurotransmitter adenosine, which promotes sleep and reduces anxious behavior.

People with Mood Disorders and Mental Illness

The typical Western diet, which is high in processed foods, sugars and other carbs, triggers biological processes that induce mood disorders like depression and anxiety. Sugar is possibly the most addictive substance on the planet, so it is little wonder that it would cause problems with mood. Many people rely on antidepressants and other medications to deal with their mood disorders; however, they can also be treated naturally. Eliminating sugar is the first step. Following a ketogenic diet can dramatically improve mood.

Additionally, the neurological processes stimulated by a ketogenic diet can treat more severe mental illnesses, such as bipolar and schizophrenia. While going keto is unlikely to cure the disease, it can help to manage symptoms.

It is important to remember that mood disorders and mental illnesses are multifaceted and can be triggered by stressful events and other environmental factors; they also seem to have a genetic link. While improving the brain's chemistry, a ketogenic diet is unable to resolve these other factors that contribute to mental illness and mood disorders.

Depression:
As opposed to sadness, which is a normal emotion that everyone experiences; depression is a clinical condition in which a lowered mood persists for weeks, months and even years. It results in a severely lowered quality of life both for the depressed individual and his or her family.

21

Numerous case studies exist to support the idea that a ketogenic diet can help treat depression and these case studies seem to be backed by scientific evidence and data. One cause of depression is neurotoxicity spurred by imbalances of the neurotransmitters GABA and glutamate. The use of ketones is able to improve the balance, thereby alleviating some of the chemical causes of depression.

Additionally, depression and inflammation are strongly linked. Conditions such as leaky gut syndrome, which is becoming more prevalent among Westerners eating a high-carb diet, decimate the microbiome of the gut, which is responsible for much of the hormones that the body produces. This alone can lead to the chemical imbalances that are associated with depression. Leaky gut syndrome and a less-than-optimal microbiome also contribute to inflammation, which can also cause or worsen depression. The ketogenic diet eliminates the foods that lead to intestinal problems, making it ideal to treat some of the causes of depression.

Adapting a ketogenic diet is just one aspect of overcoming depression and it is not a substitute for counseling.

Anxiety:

While some stress is beneficial and necessary for daily function, anxiety refers to a large amount of stress that hampers a person to complete the tasks he or she needs to do and lowers the overall quality of life. The build-up of stress hormones, such as cortisol and adrenaline, can cause stressful events to affect a person's metabolic processes. In addition to depression, anxiety-related disorders are on the rise, especially in children, who are constantly expected to achieve increasingly high expectations. The high-sugar diet adopted by many Westerners is known to contribute to anxiety and also fuels the release of cortisol and adrenaline. Eliminating sugar and exercising regularly are important to reducing levels of stress hormones. The ketogenic diet can also help stabilize the metabolic processes that lead to anxiety and reverse the damage caused by it.

As with depression, there are numerous case studies of people who suffered from anxiety and experienced substantial relief from following a ketogenic diet. This is possible because the metabolic processes in the brain are transformed through the creation and burning of ketones for energy instead of using sugar.

Schizophrenia:

Schizophrenia is a rare but serious mental illness in which a person experiences things that are not present as if they are happening. They typically experience hallucinations, which are not limited to seeing things that are not present but can also include hearing things (the "voices" associated with schizophrenia) and feeling sensations, such as itching, that do not have a physical cause. The exact causes are not known, but there seem to be both genetic and environmental factors. Treatment for schizophrenia includes behavior modification therapy and heavy medication regimens.

People suffering from schizophrenia are at a high risk of suicide and also of harming others; many need full-time care throughout their entire lives. In laboratory trials, mice whose brains were induced to have the same chemical structure as a schizophrenic brain and who had schizophrenic behaviors were fed a ketogenic diet. After three weeks, some of their mental processes became completely normal. While there is presently no data to support the treatment of schizophrenic humans with a ketogenic diet, there is certainly promise.

Bipolar:

Bipolar is a serious mental illness in which a person swings from periods of depression to mania. Intense manic periods can cause the person to become completely detached from reality and engage in risky behaviors that he or she would not ordinarily consider. There is a high rate of suicide and other harmful behaviors associated with bipolar disorder and while some people with bipolar are able to function on their own, others need lifelong care.

Many bipolar medications are also used to treat epilepsy. Because of the ketogenic diet's success in treating epilepsy, researchers were interested to find if it could also treat bipolar. Scientific evidence says that yes, it may be able to. Seizure medications that reduce the amount of sodium in the extracellular area are the only ones that are effective at treating bipolar; the ketogenic diet is effective at achieving the same thing.

Sodium is responsible for many of the metabolic processes that occur within the brain, as keeping an optimal balance of sodium and potassium is necessary for ensuring the correct electrical function that enables communication between neurons. Whacked-out sodium levels can cause problems with the functioning of neurons, which can trigger the psychotic episodes associated with bipolar. This is the reason why bipolar medication seeks to stabilize the brain's sodium.

By helping the brain maintain optimal sodium levels, both within neurons and outside of them, the ketogenic diet is able to achieve the same effect as bipolar medication.

People with Cerebral Palsy

Cerebral palsy is a neurological condition that is usually caused by lack of oxygen during birth or during the first five years of life. The brain damage caused by the lack of oxygen can lead to problems including seizures, lack of coordination, muscle spasms, difficulty with depth perception, speech difficulties and hearing and vision problems. There is no cure for cerebral palsy, but a ketogenic diet can be part of a treatment plan to improve the quality of life for people who have it.

The ketogenic can be hugely effective at treating the seizures that are associated with cerebral palsy. Further research into how it can help other aspects of cerebral palsy, such as brain damage and muscle spasms, is necessary to see how effective it is as a global treatment.

People Who Want To Lose Weight

The body's chemistry, not the arithmetic of calories in versus calories out, is what determines whether people gain weight or lose weight. Consuming carbs leads to the production of insulin, which turns on the body's fat-producing hormones. Research is increasingly finding that insulin is directly related to weight gain. Unless you immediately burn off the sugars that you consume, they will be stored as fat. This occurs regardless of whether you are eating "diet" foods or not. The key to losing weight is not in restricting calories but in lowering your insulin levels.

People on the ketogenic diet often find that they lose weight without having to restrict calories. They feel less hungry, have a much more stable appetite and feel more satisfied after eating. Without sugar being used as the body's primary fuel source, they immediately begin to burn through fat.

Some doctors have suggested that people on the ketogenic diet immediately begin to lose water weight rather than actual fat. However, this claim comes back to the faulty reasoning about the body needing carbs for energy in the form of glucose. The ketogenic diet leads the body to respond as if it is in a state of fasting by burning through fat at a high rate.

People with Fatty Liver Disease

The liver is an organ that is part of the digestive system; it filters out toxins, synthesizes enzymes and other chemicals necessary for digestion, breaks down carbs and even helps with blood clotting! It is a very important organ and keeping it healthy is of the utmost importance. Fatty liver disease is the first in a progression of liver problems. One type is caused by alcohol consumption and the other type is correlated with genetics, obesity, cholesterol and consumption of carbohydrates. Symptoms include fatigue, weight loss, nausea, confusion, lack of clarity and overall weakness. Left untreated, it could turn into cirrhosis or scarring of the liver. Cirrhosis is a serious disease that causes fluids to accumulate throughout the body, muscles to atrophy, internal bleeding, liver failure and jaundice.

While alcohol-based fatty liver disease is treated by completely abstaining from alcohol, non-alcoholic fatty liver disease (NAFLD) can be treated through diet. Adopting a high-fat diet seems to be counter-intuitive for treating a disease characterized by the fat build-up in the liver; carbs are actually more often the culprit behind NAFLD. People with NAFLD who adopt the ketogenic diet have shown reductions in the fats in their livers and overall better liver function.

If you have NAFLD and want to get on the ketogenic diet, make sure you inform your doctor. He or she may recommend frequent testing to monitor how the diet is affecting your liver.

People with Acne

Acne is a skin condition that results from unbalanced hormones, especially insulin and cortisol. Insulin causes the creation of new skin cells and causes them to stick together, both of which can lead to breakouts. It also stimulates the production of sebum, which is a type of oil the skin produces and testosterone, which also causes acne.

Severely reducing insulin levels by following a ketogenic diet has been shown to drastically help people who suffer from acne. The thought of following a high-fat diet to decrease the skin's oil production seems counterintuitive, but again, it all comes back to the body's complex chemistry and metabolism.

Many people find that when they first begin the ketogenic diet, their acne actually gets worse. However, this is usually because hormone levels are stabilizing and inflammation is healing. A month or so in, acne begins to heal and, with time, even the scars begin to go away.

People with ADD, ADHD and Executive Dysfunctions

ADD, or attention deficit disorder and ADHD, attention deficit and hyperactive disorder, cause many children and adults to have difficulty focusing and staying on task. While some people think of the disorders as people just not being willing to sit still and be quiet, they are actually rooted in neurological processes that involve neurotransmitters and other aspects of the brain's chemistry. They are often treated with medication, although some people prefer to treat them through lifestyle and forego medication. Executive function disorders are common in people with ADD and ADHD. Think of all of the functions that an executive at an office must perform: delegate tasks to employees, manage a busy schedule, coordinate meetings, oversee various departments, etc. Imagine an office trying to function without an executive and all of the different parts are running but not being coordinated. That is what an executive function disorder looks like. People with an executive function disorder know what they need to do, but they are unable to figure out exactly how to carry out the tasks.

The ketogenic diet can be of benefit to people struggling with these disorders. Parents of children with these disorders usually restrict sugar intake, as it can lead to an increase in symptoms. Consumption of whole foods without any preservatives can help decrease symptoms, as can eating high levels of healthy fats. While there haven't been many clinical trials done regarding the benefits of the ketogenic diet for ADD, ADHD and executive function disorders, there are numerous case studies suggesting that it can be very helpful.

People with a History of Eating Disorders

Eating disorders are not primarily physical but rather psychiatric problems. They tend to have deep roots in self-image, self-esteem, self-confidence and social wellbeing. The most common eating disorder is anorexia, a condition in which sufferers have an irrational fear of weight gain and see themselves as much larger than they actually are. They starve themselves and as a result, have severe nutrient deficiencies and are severely underweight. Left untreated, anorexics can die from the disorder. People with anorexia typically have an intense fear of fat, even though carbs are much more of a culprit in terms of weight gain. Because they are in a state of starvation (as opposed to fasting), they crave sweets and may binge eat on fat-free carbs. Eating a high-fat diet is not a good idea for someone who has been struggling with anorexia.

Additionally, because it promotes weight loss, anorexics should avoid it. Another common eating disorder is bulimia, a condition in which someone binge eats and then induces either vomiting or diarrhea to rid the body of all of the calories consumed. The severe instability that the body faces can make the ketogenic diet quite dangerous. However, if done under the careful supervision of a physician and psychiatrist, people with bulimia can find that the ketogenic diet is actually very healing for both their minds and their bodies. This must be done as part of a comprehensive treatment program and not a method of losing weight (as a substitute for purging).

People with Gallbladder Problems

People with gallbladder problems or with no gallbladder should avoid the ketogenic diet because they have difficulty processing fats. The gallbladder stores bile, a chemical that helps break down fats in the intestines. With the decreased levels of bile, the fat is unable to be absorbed and a nutrient deficiency results. Additionally, the ketogenic diet can lead to gallstones, which can exacerbate existing gallbladder problems.

However, under a doctor's careful supervision, people with gallbladder issues can take some steps to enable them to follow the ketogenic diet successfully. Consuming foods that stimulate the production of bile and optimal levels of stomach acid, such as ginger, celery, cucumbers, apple cider vinegar, artichokes, asparagus and dandelion greens can help avoid some of the problems with fat absorption. Drinking plenty of water — four cups within the first hour of waking up and an additional four cups before lunch — is essential. This will mean a lot of trips to the bathroom, so you will have to decide if your lifestyle will allow you to follow the ketogenic diet with gallbladder issues.

People Who Have Had Bariatric Surgery

After having stomach-altering surgery, such as a gastric bypass, the ketogenic diet can prove to be challenging. People who have had bariatric surgery have usually struggled with morbid obesity for much of their lives and have spent just as much time trying out different diets in the attempt to lose weight. The problem is that when they are successful at losing weight, they are equally successful at gaining it back.

While the ketogenic diet provides the benefit of weight loss, it is not primarily a weight-loss tool. When people who have been on the ketogenic diet revert back to eating a moderate amount of carbs, they tend to gain back some of the weight that they lose. For someone who has had bariatric surgery, this means getting back onto the weight-loss, weight-gain roller coaster. The results can be demoralizing, especially after so much effort was put into the weight-loss surgery.

Instead, people who have had bariatric surgery are usually advised to follow a modified ketogenic diet, which allows for a high protein intake rather than a high fat intake. If you have had bariatric surgery, consult with your physician about how you can get your body into a state of ketosis without getting back onto the weight-loss, weight-gain roller coaster.

People with Kidney Problems

While the ketogenic diet is unlikely to cause harmful effects for people who don't have kidney problems, those who have pre-existing issues are more likely to experience complications. Your kidneys are the organs that filter your blood and remove toxins and other waste products to be excreted as urine. You only need one functioning kidney to live, but people who have a history of kidney problems tend to have an issue with both.

Diets that are high in protein tend to be harder on the kidneys because they cause them to work more to excrete the excess calcium, potassium, sodium and by-products of metabolizing proteins. The process of ketosis can cause kidney stones to form and also causes the blood to become more acidic, leading to potential complications for those with a kidney condition. Left untreated, kidney problems can lead to a need for dialysis, a time-consuming and taxing procedure in which the blood is artificially filtered a few times each week.

If you have pre-existing kidney problems but want to follow the ketogenic diet, consult with your doctor and only change your diet under his or her supervision. You may need to be monitored and tested frequently to ensure that the diet is not harming your kidneys.

People Who Are Underweight

While obesity is the primary factor behind many chronic diseases and is reaching epidemic proportions, there are many people who are actually underweight. This may be because of metabolic problems, such as hyperthyroidism, an intense exercise regimen, or not consuming enough calories to meet the body's nutritional needs. There could also be serious underlying health problems, especially if a person with a normal weight begins to lose weight without making any lifestyle changes. Unexpected weight loss can signal serious problems, including diabetes and cancer.

The ketogenic diet is known to induce weight loss, so even though it is much healthier than many other diets, it can have a negative effect on people who are already underweight. If you are underweight and want to begin the ketogenic diet for its health benefits, speak with your doctor. He or she may advise that you adopt a modified ketogenic diet, which will include more carbs and protein to help you gain weight while eating more foods that will induce ketosis.

People Who Should Avoid the Ketogenic Diet

If you are under any medication, breastfeeding, or have any degenerative disease, please see a doctor who understands the ketogenic diet. Your health could be aggravated due to your condition. The ketogenic diet is for the purposes of improving your health and not making things worse. It's better to be safe and consult your doctor than be sorry about it just because you failed to have a consultation.

Chapter Two:
Understanding the Keto Diet

T o understand how the keto diet works, you must first know how your body converts the food that you eat into energy and how it uses it. This is done by your digestive system through digestion. Digestion is the process of breaking down food through mechanical and chemical actions. Without breaking down food into their simpler forms, your body cannot use it for energy, growth and cell repair. The food that you eat consists of nutrients that can be primarily divided into two classifications: macronutrients and micronutrients. While micronutrients help our body to repair, grow and protect itself, macronutrients provide the energy our body needs. These two nutrient subdivisions could be further divided - the macronutrients into fats, proteins and carbohydrates; and micronutrients into the vast array of vitamins and minerals.

Carbohydrates

Carbohydrates come from sugars, starches and fiber found in the fruit, grains and vegetables that you eat. These are broken down by the saliva in your mouth, small intestine and pancreas into glucose, sucrose and fructose (simple sugars). The simple sugars are for the body's immediate energy needs.

Protein

Proteins come from meat, eggs and beans that you eat. These are all broken down by the stomach, small intestines and pancreas into amino acids.

These are used by your body to create neurotransmitters, non-essential amino acids and other protein-based compounds. Excess amino acids are circulated and used to repair damaged tissues or are stored as glucose.

Fats

Fats come from oils and fat in our diet. These are broken down by the liver and pancreas into fatty acids and glycerol. These are used by the body to repair cells and make different chemicals or tissues.

Vitamins

Vitamins come from the food solids and liquid that you eat. As these are broken down by your system, the small and large intestines absorb the vitamins for use in different body functions, from fighting inflammation to repairing cell damage. These are all absorbed in the small intestines by specialized cells that pass across the intestinal lining. Your bloodstream circulates amino acids, simple sugars, glycerol and other salts and vitamins to your liver. The vessels that move white blood cells and lymph throughout the body, called as lymphatic system, circulates fatty acids and vitamins.

This whole process of digestion is controlled by your nervous system and the hormones your body produce. Your nerves cause muscles of the GI tract to contract or relax to digest food and release a substance to control the movement of food and the production of digestive juices. Your hormones, on the other hand, regulate appetite and stimulate the production of digestive juices.

There will be excess nutrients that your body won't need after this whole ordeal. Your excess blood sugar and amino acids would be stored in your body as either glycogen in liver, muscle and fat cells. The excess amino acids get stored as glucose while the excess fats get stored as triglycerides in the fat cells. Vitamins in excess are either expelled through urine, if water-soluble, or stored in the liver and fat cells, if fat-soluble.

The Fasted State

Around 2 to 8 hours after your last meal, your body enters a state of fasting. In this state, your body's blood sugar drops to a lower threshold level, which also brings down the levels of insulin in it. With the drop of glucose in your blood, a hormone from the liver, called glucagon is released to release the stored energy in your cells. This raises your glucose levels in your bloodstream, which is primarily used by the brain and red blood cells.

After these stores are used up, the body starts to be in a state of ketosis. Triglycerides are released from fat cells and are used by your muscles and liver cells as fuel. From the liver's use of triglycerides, ketones are formed and used if more energy is needed. As your body's fasted state goes further, more triglycerides are released, broken down and used for energy. As you can see, thanks to ketosis, the body can freely switch energy consumption from blood sugar to the stored glycogen, glucose and triglycerides. However, due to the high carbohydrate diets, your body had somehow gotten used to only using blood sugar for energy.

Whenever it goes down, you start getting hungry and craving for a meal with carbohydrates. If you do eat a meal without carbohydrates, you don't feel as satisfied. This does not normally occur when ketosis occurs in a fasted state due to the ketones that prevent hunger hormones from coming out and trigger hormones that signal your brain to feel sated as if you ate a meal.

Ketosis Effect

On a diet that is high or centered around carbohydrates, your body is primarily burning glucose for fuel. Since it is frequently supplied with carbohydrates through your meals, it does not adapt itself out of a glucose burning state and into fat burning. And whenever it needs more glucose, your body would just tell you that it's time to eat. As any excess in caloric intake would result in your body storing fat, it would just keep storing fat whenever you do. Since it is in a standard state of using glucose as a primary source of energy, your body won't readily use what is in its fat stores. This perpetuates a cycle of your body gaining fat from the excess caloric intake and being unable to burn it for energy.

With a ketogenic diet, the body does not primarily depend on carbohydrates for your body's daily caloric requirements. This results in your body adapting to this diet and, then naturally, switching to looking for its required energy and primarily using fat for fuel. With your body in a state of ketosis, it uses up your fat stores more readily whenever your body runs out of the fat it got from your last meal. Instead of you feeling hungry, it just uses up the stored energy in your body fat.

There are two ways that you can do for your body to achieve a state of ketosis. This is through fasting from food or substituting the carbohydrates in your diet with healthy fats, which is what the ketogenic diet does. Since fasting in the long-term is not a sustainable way to achieve ketosis, the ketogenic diet is the way to go for anyone who wants to take advantage of this fat burning state of your body. However, the ketogenic diet goes beyond the ratio of the carbohydrates, proteins and fats that are in your meals. You must eat the right nutrients to be able to healthily achieve ketosis. Doing so otherwise could lead to chronic inflammation, metabolic disorders and other degenerative diseases.

Chapter Three:
Benefits of Keto Diet

The ketogenic diet is absolutely unique and it gives you benefits that you wouldn't find in any other diet. The main aim behind the diet is to reduce your dependence on carbohydrates and inducing your body to burn more fats.

Fighting Cancer

The ketogenic diet is a natural deterrent for cancer cells. The ketogenic diet usually consists of 75 percent fat, 20 percent protein and 5 percent carbohydrates. This limits the number of carbs and sugar that you consume. Cancer cells replicate themselves throughout your body once they start growing. These cells need sugar in order to create enough energy to replicate themselves. Since the ketogenic diet eliminates intake of sugar, the cancer cells are left stranded.

The diet also reduces your intake of carbohydrates. This further helps in fighting cancer, as the cancer cells do not have an alternative source to generate energy. This does not mean that you won't have the energy that you need for daily activities. Your regular cells can use fats to generate energy but cancer cells cannot simply switch to a different source.

Helps in Weight Loss

If we consume carbohydrates, insulin is released throughout the body in order to increase blood glucose. Insulin is a type of hormone. Its basic function is to ensure that the body has enough energy for all of its needs. So, when insulin is released it further propagates the cells to save as much energy as possible. The cells initially save the energy in the form of glycogen (carbohydrates in their stored form) then later on as fat.

The ketogenic diet aims at reducing the level of carbohydrates that you consume so that they are almost negligible in your body. This prevents your body from releasing insulin. When insulin is not released in the body then there is a lack of glycogen, which the body needs in order to generate energy. Your body is forced to burn fats in order to generate energy. This helps in reducing the number of fats that are stored in your body and therefore, helps you to lose weight.

Treating Alzheimer's disease

Alzheimer is a disease that slowly deteriorates your nervous system. If it goes untreated it can even lead to Dementia. The ketogenic diet is the perfect way to treat Alzheimer's.

When you get old, the nervous system stops working properly and tends to slow down after a while. This causes mood swings, random episodes of dementia and most importantly memory loss. To prevent Alzheimer's from growing, it's important to take care of your nervous system.

The nervous system is directly linked to the brain. So, to help the brain it is important to consume healthy fats. Healthy fats make your brain more active. The ketogenic diet consists of 70 percent healthy fats and therefore it helps the brain.

Lower Blood Pressure

Elevated blood pressure can lead to many diseases including heart attack, kidney failure and others.

The ketogenic diet makes sure that you do not consume too many carbs. This reduces the blood pressure of your body. It's been seen in numerous cases that a reduction in consumption of carbs led to decreased blood pressure. The reason behind this is that a low carb diet induces the body to store fewer fluids. This includes the constituent fluids present in the blood.

A lower blood pressure reduces the risk of an early death and also makes you feel more energetic than before.

Improved brain function

The idea that the brain functions entirely on glucose is simply untrue. The brain only needs about 40 grams of glucose per day (that level may vary according to the individual), which can be synthesized from proteins through the process of gluconeogenesis. Once the body becomes fully adapted to the ketogenic diet, the brain can meet 75% of its energy needs from ketones, with the remaining 25% coming from the glucose made from proteins.

The brain actually contains astrocytes, which produce ketones. This fact indicates that the brain actually does function more optimally on ketones. Also, the fact that the ketogenic diet was originally established to treat neurological disorders, especially epilepsy, shows how important they are to establishing optimal brain function.

Ketones are actually a more efficient fuel for the brain and create fewer waste products than glucose.

Over time, the brain clears out all of the waste products generated by relying on glucose for energy. Running on ketones, it is able to establish optimal sodium levels between neurons, thereby decreasing the symptoms of diseases like depression, anxiety, schizophrenia and bipolar. Damaged neurons can begin to heal and even regenerate. Thoughts become clearer, mood increases and the brain operates optimally.

Improved nutrition

Without eating many fruit and limiting the vegetables consumed, one concern about the ketogenic diet is that over time, it can lead to nutrient deficiencies. While it may be beneficial in the short term to help achieve weight loss and other health goals, over the long term, it can be harmful because it does not provide complete nutrition. The only thing necessary to induce ketosis is very few carbs and lots of fat. This can be accomplished by drinking canola oil (which is not natural at all, as there is no such thing as a canola plant), eating margarine (which is made from trans fats) and pushing down hot dogs. Eating like this will certainly create severe nutrient deficiencies and cause illness.

However, a proper approach to the ketogenic diet, which includes lots of fatty cuts from high-quality meat produced from animals that are raised organically, nuts, leafy green vegetables, dairy, butter, olive oil and avocados, the diet is actually very nutrient dense. In fact, you will be consuming much more vitamins and minerals than in a typical American diet.

Lower cholesterol and risk of heart disease

The scary fact behind heart disease is that it is caused by eating carbs, not fats. Increasing research is revealing that heart disease rates are higher in people who eat a lot of carbs, even though traditional advice is that people with risk factors for heart disease should limit their fat intake. Carbs raise blood triglycerides, the dangerous fats that float through your bloodstream and can cause blockages when they build up to dangerous levels. Additionally, growing evidence suggests that carbs, not fats, raise the bad LDL cholesterol that can also clog arteries. The more carbs you eat, the higher your risk of heart disease.

There is a lot of misunderstanding about how cholesterol actually works. It is necessary for bodily function and is produced naturally; the body's cholesterol levels are actually affected very little by the foods that we eat. The carriers of the cholesterol are either the high-density lipoproteins (HDL) or low-density lipoproteins (LDL), which are determined by the foods that we eat. Eating a lot of cholesterol doesn't increase chances of heart disease.

Triglycerides are the fats that are stored in your fat cells but can also accumulate in the bloodstream. They can also accumulate in the liver, leading to fatty liver disease. They are produced from glucose, so the best way to lower your triglycerides is to severely restrict the carbs that you are consuming. Numerous studies show that a high-fat diet, as compared with a high-carb diet, is very effective at lowering levels of triglycerides, as long as the fats consumed are healthy.

Healthy fats actually purge the bad triglycerides and LDL from your bloodstream, thereby lowering the risk factors for heart disease. They clean up the blood

Increased energy

Insulin, which is secreted whenever carbs are consumed so that cells are able to absorb the energy, causes fatigue and drowsiness. This is why you often feel sleepy after eating a large meal. Additionally, glucose is not very efficient at creating energy and leaves a lot of waste products, thereby exacerbating fatigue. People on carb-rich diets tend to sleep much more than people on high-fat diets because they just don't have energy.

Once insulin levels are lowered and the body is adjusted to burning ketones instead of glucose, energy levels increase dramatically. Some people on the ketogenic diet report needing less sleep and are able to thrive on just six hours, whereas doctors recommend seven to eight. Interestingly, traditional cultures that consume high-fat diets also sleep closer to six hours, suggesting that there may be a link between eating a high-fat diet and needing less sleep.

Balanced hormones

At the heart of many diseases are imbalanced hormones. Insulin is one of the most proliferate hormones in the human body and problems with its levels immediately affect other hormones, including sex hormones, satiety hormones and hunger hormones. Stabilizing and permanently lowering insulin levels leads to balanced hormones all across the body. This is why people with metabolic syndrome, PCOS, acne and other hormonal problems benefit immensely from the ketogenic diet.

Decreased inflammation

Inflammation is the body's natural response to infection and foreign invaders. When you cut your finger, the skin around the cut quickly becomes red and inflamed, as your body is responding to the microbes that may be entering. While some inflammation is good as an acute response, many people live in a state of chronic inflammation caused by poor diet. Inflamed tissues can develop scar tissue and be unable to function properly. Inflamed joints become painful and inflamed blood vessels cause heart disease.

A ketogenic diet has been shown to substantially decrease inflammation over the long term. The body is still able to use inflammation as an acute response to foreign invaders, but it is no longer a chronic issue.

Chapter Four:
Basics of Planning Meals

To know what you have to eat on a ketogenic diet, you will have to understand caloric requirements and content and fats, protein and carbohydrates. You have to understand their different kinds and the different roles they perform for your body. Furthermore, you need to know what macronutrients are good and harmful for your health so that you can build a diet that is both ketogenic and healthy.

In addition, for the ketogenic diet to work, you need to remove all packaged and processed foods from your diet. It should consist of high-quality, healthy fats, fiber-rich carbohydrates with the least net carbohydrates (total carbohydrates minus fiber) as possible.

Important: Before you create a plan for your ketogenic diet, you need to consult first a nutritionist or a medical professional to determine the number of daily calories you require based on your age, height, weight, gender and age as well as body fat percentage. This would make sure that you are not merely guessing in setting the calories you need for your body.
Fats

In the 1980s, doctors, nutritionists and public health officials campaigned to the public that fats are not a part of a healthy diet. They said that fat is the cause of weight gain and heart disease. However, this is only true for the bad quality of fat in food. Fats play a critical role in providing a denser caloric content per gram compared to proteins and carbohydrates. Because of this, fat can provide adequate energy when food is scarce or when a person is unable to consume large amounts of food.

Fats

Fats in your diet contain mixtures of fatty acids. These nutrients contain a mixture of saturated and unsaturated fats. Saturated fats are most abundant in animal-derived fats while unsaturated fats are most abundant in plant-derived ones. Other than the dense caloric property fats, it provides fatty acids that regulate inflammation in the body. It carries fat-soluble vitamins. Lastly, it provides texture and flavor to your meal, making it more satisfying to your appetite.

Fats to avoid
Excess Saturated Fat

The key to having healthy fat consumption is to minimize the consumption of food rich in saturated fats. Although your body needs both kinds of fat, saturated fats from foods derived from plants are enough to provide you with your saturated fat needs. Having high levels of saturated fat in your body leads to heart and cardiovascular disease.

Moreover, it is not enough to replace saturated fat-rich foods with fat-free food products as these are high in carbohydrates and increase the risk of the same disease mentioned. Here's a list of foods rich in saturated fat that you should avoid:

- Fat from processed meats like sausages, ham and burgers

- Fatty meat
- Hard cheeses
- Butter
- Lard
- Ghee
- Palm Oil

Trans Fat

Trans fat, or trans-unsaturated fats, occur in nature albeit in small amounts, but they are also widely manufactured commercially from vegetable fats for use in various manufactured food products. This is created by adding hydrogen gas to vegetable oil, which causes the oil to become solid at room temperature.

The reason why food manufacturers create and use this is to make food have a longer shelf life or have a better flavor. These fats contribute to insulin resistance and unbalance your cholesterol levels by increasing the bad and decreasing the good.

Manufactured trans-fat can be found in food products like:

- Baked goods like cake, pie crusts and crackers and ready-made frosting
- Snacks like packaged microwave popcorn and potato, corn and tortilla chips.
- Fried food due to the oil used in the cooking process
- Refrigerator dough like canned biscuits, cinnamon rolls and frozen pizza crusts
- Non-dairy coffee creamer
- Margarine
- In food labels, trans fat can also be listed as shortening, hydrogenated oil, partially hydrogenated oil and hydrogenated vegetable oil.

Fats you can eat

The key to having a healthy ketogenic diet is choosing wisely the fats you include in your diet without exceeding your calorie requirement. The important part of this diet is to consume the correct ratio of macronutrients. You need between five and ten percent of your calories to be from net carbs, 15 and 30 percent from protein and 65 to 75 percent or more from fat to be able to benefit from the ketones that get produced by the liver.

Is there a right amount of fat intake with a ketogenic diet? This amount will vary for everybody. It depends on your goals. You don't need to count your calories or fat intake on a keto diet since eating foods that are naturally low in carbs keep your feeling full longer.

Studies have shown that fats and proteins are the most filling nutrients and carbs are the least. Fats contribute to a steady energy supply and don't cause insulin spikes. This is the reason you don't have cravings, mood swings or fluctuating energy. For some, counting calories and tracking macros can help break through a stubborn weight loss plateau.

The macronutrient ratio isn't all you need to consider. You need to understand what fats are good for you and what can be detrimental to your health. The different qualities and types of fat make a difference. When figuring out what fats and oil to use, here are some simple rules to follow:

When cooking, use saturated fats. These fats have gotten a bad rap as being bad for us. We have heard that cholesterol and saturated fats cause obesity and heart disease for the past 50 years. This lipid hypothesis was created by Ancel Keys' fraudulent and flawed research. Saturated fats can be found in palm oil, coconut oil, eggs, tallow, lard, ghee, butter, cream and red meat. These oils have a high smoke point, long shelf life and are the most stable. Use these for cooking. The majority of fats need to come from monounsaturated and saturated fats.

Try adding medium chain triglycerides to your diet. These are fats that can be easily digested. These triglycerides can be found in coconut oil. They act differently when ingested and are sent straight to the liver. They can be immediately used for energy. They are found in palm oil and butter in lesser quantities. Medium chain triglycerides are used by bodybuilders and athletes to improve their performance and help them lose fat. If your body is able to handle pure MCT oil without causing any stomach problems, you should be able to find it as a supplement.

Include monounsaturated fatty acids. Omega 9, oleic acid or monounsaturated fatty acids can be found in nuts, beef, olives and avocados. These help to prevent heart disease. Consuming monounsaturated fatty acids can give better serum lipid profiles. Monounsaturated fatty acids like macadamia nut, avocado and extra virgin olive oil are the best for using cold like drizzling over a finished a meal.

You can use unsaturated fats. You do not heat them. Our body needs omega 6s, Omega 3s and polyunsaturated fatty acids. These are common in our everyday lives and we consume too many. These fatty acids are called poly because they have many double bonds. When these bonds are heated, they react with oxygen to form compounds that are harmful like free radicals. This process increases inflammation and makes free radicals that put us at risk for cancer and heart disease. Polyunsaturated fats are not stable and should not be used for high heat cooking. Avocado oil, flaxseed oil, sesame oil, nut oils and extra virgin olive oil are best to use cold. Flaxseed oil shouldn't be heated and needs to be refrigerated. Olive, Macadamia and avocado oil can be used for light cooking or for finishing the meal.

The Omega 6 fatty acids and omega 3 fatty acids need to be balanced. Both of these are polyunsaturated fatty acids and are essential. Studies have shown that most diets are deficient in omega 3s. The omega 6 and omega 3 ratio is unfavorable between 15 to 1 and 17 to 1. This ratio needs to be balanced at one to one. It will be better for your health if you can get this ratio as close to one to one as possible. Studies have shown that eating more omega 6 and lower omega 3s are known to cause inflammatory diseases, autoimmune disorders, stroke and cardiovascular disease. Reducing your intake of omega 6s might protect you against these diseases. You are probably getting enough omega 6s so try to focus on increasing the intake of omega 3s by eating macadamia nuts, walnuts, grass-fed meat, fermented cod liver oil and wild salmon.

Your Omega 3 intake should come from animals. Omega 3 is either long chain that is found in seafood and fish or short chain that is found in nuts and seeds. While Eicosapentaenoic acid or EPA and docosahexaenoic acid or DHA affect omega 6s to 3s ratios, the alpha-linoleic acid or ALA needs to be converted to DHA or EPA. Our bodies can't convert ALA to DHA or EPA. This is why you need to get the omega 3s from the meat of animals. When buying meat, find grass fed to get the most omega 3s. Meat from animals that have been grain fed had very low omega 3s but packed full of omega 6s.

Be aware of shelf life, oxidation rate and smoke point. A higher smoke point is better. Oils that have a high smoke point can be used to cook foods at high temperatures. If you heat the oil above its smoke point, this can damage the oil and release free radicals.

Having an oxidation rate that is slow is better. The oxidation rate increases when it gets heated to its smoking point. These can also oxidize on the shelf. Metals like copper and iron can also cause them to oxidize. Any oil is capable of going rancid while sitting on in the pantry. This will load them with free radicals. Higher saturated fat oils will last longer around 12 to 24 months. Oils that are high in monounsaturated fats will last about six to twelve months. Polyunsaturated fats have a shelf life of about two to six months.

Stay away from all unhealthy oils. Corn, grapeseed, soybean, canola, cottonseed, safflower, sunflower oils, trans fats, partially hydrogenated oils, hydrogenated oils, margarine and processed vegetable oils are all bad for your health. Processed oils and trans fatty acids:

- Are oxidized with high heat and created free radicals.
- These are created from genetically modified seeds.
- Are pro-inflammatory and bad for your gut.
- Eating trans fats raises the risk of developing coronary heart disease.

- Consuming trans fats will affect cholesterol levels negatively. They reduce the level of HDL or good cholesterol and increase the level of LDL or bad cholesterol.
- Can cause an increased risk of cancer.

All of these fats exist within nature and occur during the processing of polyunsaturated fatty acids in food production. These naturally occurring trans fats are beneficial when you compare them to artificial trans fats. These natural trans fats can be found in the meat of animals that have been grass fed and dairy products.

Metabolic poison refers to artificial trans fats. Get these out of your diet by staying away from any food that contains partially hydrogenated or hydrogenated oils. You can find these in French fries, crackers, cookies and margarine.

Proteins

Most foods contain some amount of protein including vegetables and grain. Foods that have substantial amounts of protein are meat from animals, dairy products, beans and nuts. It can provide energy for your body. However, it is not its primary purpose.

When broken down into amino acids, the body would use this to create its own proteins intended for various purposes. With the 20 amino acids that your body would need, it can create an infinite number of proteins like enzymes for chemical reactions, hormones for triggering organs, collagen for bone structure and antibodies for the immune system. Your body's proteins are constantly broken down and re-synthesized to build more proteins. Most of the amino acids from broken down protein are reused, but some are lost and must be replaced through your diet.

Proteins to avoid

What you have to watch out for in proteins in your diet is eating too much of it. The excess protein that you got from your food would be converted to sugar and then fat which would be stored for later use. It could also increase the stimulation of your mTOR, which increases your chances of developing cancer. Additionally, the excess protein requires your body to remove more nitrogen, a by-product of protein digestion, which stresses out your kidneys.

Proteins to eat

Moderate consumption of high-quality protein is the key. Protein for a ketogenic diet should come from a variety of plant and animal sources. Meat products should be lean to avoid adding fats that are mostly saturated. The suggested protein for a ketogenic diet varies from person to person. Generally, the recommended daily protein of 0.8g per pound of lean body mass for a sedentary lifestyle, 0.8 to 1g per pound of body mass for a lightly active lifestyle and 1.0 – 1.2g for a highly active lifestyle.

Carbohydrates

Carbohydrates are the starches, sugars and fibers found in the food that we eat. The sugars and starches we eat are broken down into its simplest chemical forms while, as it is indigestible, fibers just pass through the digestive system.

Sugars, also known as simple carbohydrates, are found in fruit and vegetables that can be broken down to sucrose and/ or fructose. Starches, also known as complex carbohydrates, are found in grains that can be broken down into glucose (also known as blood sugar).

Of all these carbohydrates, glucose is the most preferred as it can be readily circulated from the digestive process into various parts of the body. Meanwhile, fructose can only be used for energy by the liver and sucrose is further broken down into glucose and fructose.

The role of fiber: The most common question with low carb dieters is: Do I need to include fiber when counting my carbs?

Let's see: Some soluble gets absorbed, but humans, in general, don't possess all the needed enzymes to digest fibers and then be able to get calories out of it. Because of this, fiber doesn't affect blood sugar or ketosis. You can try to get between 20 and 25 grams of net carbs or less than 50 grams of total carbs.

If the fiber isn't counted, the carbs are referred to as net carbs. Calculating net carbs can reduce how high fiber foods are impacted and allow you to eat them. This is a common argument for those who criticize the low carb diet because it lacks fiber. An important note is that fiber does not negate carbs. They are just not counted. You can't just mix some flax meal into pasta.

In Canada and the United States, food labels include fiber with the carbohydrate values in a term known as total carbs. This calculates carbs by using an indirect method. Carbs get calculated after the ash, water, fat and protein has been measured out. To figure net carbs, you subtract the amount of fiber from the total carbs. This type of food label isn't used all over the world. In Oceania, Australia and Europe, their food labels don't include fiber. They calculate carbs using a direct method. The carbs listed on their food labels will just be net carbs. Don't worry about where you buy the food but think about the country it came from.

Is there a way to be certain about the amounts of net carbs? You can follow these rules:

- Total carbs will never be less than the amount of fiber.
- The total carbs minus the fiber is never going to be less than the sugar. For example, lactose + other sugar + sugars = net carbs.
- Calories that come from carbs (without fiber) + calories that come from protein + calories that come from fat

= total kcal

Although fiber cannot be digested, it plays a key role in the digestion of carbohydrates in the body. It slows down the rate of digestion and absorption of carbohydrates, thereby preventing the blood sugar from rapidly shooting up. Aside from that, fibers provide food for your beneficial gut bacteria, improving digestion and bowel movement.

Fibers also contain phytochemicals like lycopene, lutein and indole-3-carbinol. These stimulate the immune system, fight free radicals and protect and repair the DNA.

Carbs to avoid

Refined Carbohydrates

Refined carbohydrates are whole plants or plant-derived products that have been processed to remove everything except the highly digestible carbohydrate in it. To refine carbohydrates, the whole sugar, plant, or grain is stripped of its fibers, vitamins and minerals. This is done usually as other parts of the plant cannot be digested by the body or to make the plant easier to manipulate into mixtures and food products.

Refining removes everything including valuable natural vitamins and minerals and, to circumvent the lack of micronutrients, manufacturers add synthetic vitamins and minerals back into the carbohydrates.

Refined carbohydrates in an average person's diet usually come from:

- White flour from white bread, pasta and other food products containing it.
- White rice that is usually "enriched" with the synthetic vitamins and minerals.
- Sugar from bread, pastries, sweets and breakfast cereals.
- Sugar and High Fructose Corn Syrup from sodas and other sweetened beverages.
- Sugar from any other food product that has been added before consumption like ketchup and mustard.

With the fibers removed from these carbohydrates, your body digests it quickly. This results in a rapid absorption of broken down carbohydrates into your body. Particularly, in the case of glucose, your blood sugar rises so fast that your body would have to release insulin to signal your body to start storing it. This causes a volatile and erratic volume of blood sugar in your system. This usually manifests to sluggishness and/ or hunger even though you just had a heavy carbohydrate meal. If your body experiences this often, it will pave the way for insulin resistance and, eventually, Type 2 Diabetes.

On the other hand, fructose from refined carbohydrates that are used as sweeteners and other forms of added sugars have compound said harmful effects. Excess consumption of foods containing added fructose could lead to:

- Visceral fat gain
- Increased uric acid levels leading to gout and high blood pressure,
- Insulin resistance
- Leptin resistance that disturbs body fat regulation and contributing to obesity.

High Fructose Corn Syrup

High Fructose Corn Syrup (HFCS) is a refined carbohydrate that comes from corn. It is a sugar substitute that is a hundred times sweeter than sucrose, the common sugar. Since it costs substantially less and is not affected by fluctuating import prices, it is a very good alternative for sugar. It started gaining popularity during the 1970s when it began being used by food manufacturers. Its use in different food products steadily rose since then.

The incidences of obesity are higher in countries where its use is prevalent. Add to that the fact, that in the 1980s up to the present date, obesity rates in the United States steadily rose, matching the trend of rising availability of HFCS in food products.

Moreover, studies have shown that, even in moderate consumption, HFCS is a major cause of various diseases like heart disease, obesity, cancer, dementia and liver failure. Even though HFCS is used as a substitute for sucrose, the body does not respond to it in the same way.

Carbs to Eat

In a ketogenic diet, you must stick to protein, vegetables, fats and oils, full-fat dairy and nuts and seeds of your diet. From these items, you will already be able to get the fiber that you need for your diet. Adding any kind of grain or sugar in your diet would only prevent you from reaching your goals in the diet. However, if you want to have your fix of carbohydrates, you can use flour substitutes like coconut flour and flaxseed meal.

For carbohydrates in a Standard Ketogenic Diet, the maximum daily intake is 5% of total daily calorie intake. Refer to the net carbs of the food items given in preparing the carbohydrates for your meals.

Beverages

The ketogenic diet is very particular in controlling what goes into your body. Drinking alcohol, sweetened beverages and fruit juices would mess up your sugar levels and could push you further from reaching ketosis. Therefore, you must only drink water and coffee and tea with no sweeteners, creamer and dairy. Anything else other than these three should not be drunk.

The ketogenic diet causes a natural diuretic effect. Dehydration is common for many people who are just starting on this diet. If you get bladder pain or urinary tract infections, you need to be prepared. The normal eight glasses that are recommended for you to drink - you need to drink those and then more. Our body consists of two-thirds water. Drink at least a gallon of water everyday, as hydration is extremely important.

Many choose keto friendly coffee or tea of the mornings to give their energy a boost with added fats. It is good; just remember to avoid flavored beverages as much as possible. This becomes amplified with caffeine as too much may hamper your weight loss. Try to only have about two caffeinated beverages each day.

Some examples of beverages you can have with your keto diet are:

- Water: This is your go-to for hydration. You may have sparkling or plain water.
- Broth: This is loaded with nutrients and vitamins. Most important, it gives your energy a boost by replenishing your electrolytes.
- Coffee: This will improve your mental focus and has weight loss benefits.
- Tea: This has the same effects as coffee. Some people don't like tea. Try either green or black tea.
- Almond or coconut milk: Use the unsweetened versions in a carton from your grocery store to replace your favorite dairy drink.
- Diet soda: You need to reduce or completely stop drinking these. These can cause sugar cravings and insulin spikes.
- Flavoring: These little packets are flavored with stevia or sucralose and are fine. You can also add orange, lime and lemon to your water.
- Alcohol: If you need your alcohol, choose hard liquor. Wine and beer will be too high in carbs to drink. Frequent consumption of alcohol will slow down your weight loss.

Most people like to keep themselves accountable for the actions by creating a challenge for themselves. Try using a 32-ounce water bottle and place four hair-ties around it. Every time you finish a bottle, take away one hair tie. Keep on drinking until there aren't any left.

Recommended Foods

Below is a comprehensive list of the common food items that are recommended for your ketogenic diet. Each item has information of its nutritional value arranged as such: "amount of item/ calories/fat / net carbohydrates/protein."

Protein

The best proteins for a ketogenic diet are those that are pasture-raised and grass-fed. This will minimize your exposure from bacteria and growth hormones. Choose darker poultry meat and fatty fish that are rich in omega 3. Balance out your protein portions in your meals with fats and oil to aid in its digestion.

- Ground beef (4oz, 80/ 20 / 280 / 23g / 0g / 20g)
- Ribeye steak (4oz / 330 / 25g / 0g / 27g)
- Bacon (4oz / 519 / 51g / 0g / 13g)
- Pork chop (4oz / 286 / 18g / 0g / 30g)
- Chicken thigh (4oz / 250 / 20g / 0g / 17g)
- Chicken breast (4oz / 125 / 1g / 0 / 26g)
- Salmon (4oz / 236 / 15g / 0g / 23g)
- Ground lamb (4oz / 319 / 27g / 0g / 19g)
- Liver (4oz / 135 / 5g / 0g / 19g)
- Egg (1 large / 70 / 5g / 0.5g / 6g)
- Almond butter (2tbsp / 180 / 16g / 4g/ 6)

Vegetables and Fruit

Cruciferous vegetables that are grown above ground, leafy and green are the best for a ketogenic diet. On the other hand, vegetables that grow below ground should be eaten in moderation as these have higher carbohydrate amounts.

- Cabbage (6 oz. / 43g / 0g / 6g / 2g)
- Cauliflower (6 oz. / 40 / 0g / 6g / 5g)
- Broccoli (6 oz. / 58 / 1g / 7g / 5g)
- Spinach (6 oz. / 24 / 0g / 1g / 3g)
- Romaine Lettuce (6 oz. / 29 / 1g / 2g / 2g)
- Green Bell Pepper (6 oz. / 33 / 0g / 5g / 1g)
- Baby Bella Mushrooms (6 oz. / 40 / 0g / 4g / 6g)
- Green Beans (6 oz. / 26 / 0g / 4g / 2g)
- Yellow Onion (6 oz. / 68 / 0g / 12g/ 2g)
- Blackberries (6 oz. / 73 / 1g / 8g / 2g)
- Raspberries (6 oz. / 88 / 1g / 8g / 2g)

Dairy Products

If available, give preference to raw and organic dairy products. Avoid highly processed dairy as these have a higher amount of carbohydrates than raw/ organic ones. Also avoid products with higher carbohydrate levels.

- Heavy cream (1 oz. / 100g / 12g / 0g / 0g)
- Greek yogurt (1 oz. / 28g / 1g / 1g / 3g)
- Mayonnaise (1 oz. / 180g / 20g / 0g / 0g)
- Half n' half (1 oz. / 40 / 4g / 1g / 1g)
- Cottage cheese (1 oz. / 25g / 1g / 1g / 4g)
- Cream Cheese (1 oz. / 94 / 9g / 1g / 2g)
- Mascarpone (1 oz. / 120g / 13g / 0g / 2g)
- Mozzarella (1 oz. / 70 / 5g / 1g / 5g)
- Brie (1 oz. / 95 / 8g / 0g / 6g)
- Aged Cheddar (1 oz. / 110 / 9g / 0g / 7g)

- Parmesan (1 oz. / 110 / 7g / 1g / 10g)

Nuts and Seeds

These are best when roasted to remove any anti-nutrients present. These can be added to add flavor or texture to your meals.

- Macadamia Nuts (2 oz. / 407 / 43g / 3g / 4g)
- Brazil Nuts (2 oz. / 373 / 37g / 3g / 8g)
- Pecans (2 oz. / 392 / 41g / 3g / 5g)
- Almonds (2 oz. / 328 / 28g / 5g / 12g)
- Hazelnuts (2 oz. / 356 / 36g / 3g / 9g)

Nut and Seed Flours

These can be used as a substitute for regular flour in making baked and dessert recipes.

- Almond Flour (2 oz. / 324 / 28g / 6g / 12g)
- Coconut Flour (2 oz. / 120 / 4g / 6g / 4g)
- Chia Seed Meal (2 oz. / 265 / 17g / 3g / 8g)
- Flaxseed Meal (2 oz. / 224 / 18g / 1g / 8g)
- Unsweetened Coconut (2 oz. / 445 / 40g / 8g / 4g)

Getting Started

Before you even get started on this diet, you must first decide on your goal and why you're doing this. Are you looking to lose unhealthy body fat? Are you looking to therapeutically heal a degenerative disease? Are you aiming to change your lifestyle? Whatever the case may be, you must first decide why you're going to do this diet. Without clarity on your goal, you can't choose an approach for your diet and can't properly plan for how to do it.

Get Yourself Tested

You must first determine that your body can undergo the diet and the massive adjustments it would make. You also have to determine your body fat percentage, weight and other relevant data to create your personal macronutrient mix via keto calculators available online.

Get Support

You have to talk to your family, especially if they live in the same house as you. If you're the only one who's doing this diet, your family might misunderstand when you can't eat like them, or you have a different food from theirs. Moreover, on the first few weeks, you might miss out on the next birthday party or family gathering just to distance yourself from tempting carbohydrates.

Other than that, your family can also help you in keeping you in line with the diet. They can call you out whenever you're about to slip from it. Also, if you have children, you can make it fun for them by making them your carbohydrate police at home. If you live alone, you can get support by joining community forums online.

Plan the meals that you will have

Even before you shop for your ketogenic groceries, you must first know the meals you will be eating beforehand. This would save you time and would make sure that you have the right ingredients ready for making ketogenic meals. This would reduce the excuses you can think of to just nibble on carbohydrates or say, "it would just be one meal."

Also, this gives you the opportunity to research for recipes that you might like. Other than that, after you find recipes that you like, you can plan out your meals for your next run to the grocery. Clean out the Carbohydrates out of Your House

This is the best way of preventing yourself from slipping up and "accidentally" eating that cookie. If there are no food items in your house to tempt you, you cannot be tempted to eat what you shouldn't. This would surely help you, as the first few months are the hardest due to your body still adapting to ketosis.

Undergo an Adaptation Period

To make the ketogenic diet easier for you, you could slowly ease into it by either fasting intermittently to or cut your carbohydrates. By fasting intermittently, you have 16 hours wherein you don't eat anything and only 8 hours wherein you can. This forces your body to enter a state of fasting and you get used to having your blood sugar into a fasted state.

On the other hand, by cutting your calories, your body is being trained to get used to having smaller portions of carbohydrates that it used to. Like in intermittent fasting, it decreases the shock of having very little carbohydrates in your diet. One practice is by limiting daily net carbohydrates to only 30 grams for 6 days in a week and having a high carbohydrate meal for dinner of the 7th day. This is repeated for every 7 days for at least 4 weeks.

Chapter Five:
Setting up a Plan

In this section, I will familiarize you with some practical aspects that you might need to know about to set up a plan.

Keto Shopping List

There are plenty of keto foods out there. Here is a list to help you get started with your first shopping trip:

Vegetables:

- Asparagus
- Broccoli
- Cabbage
- Pickles
- Black Olives
- Green Olives
- Sauerkraut
- Cauliflower
- Spinach, fresh and canned
- Green onions
- Iceberg Lettuce
- Mushrooms
- Okra
- Spaghetti Squash
- Yellow Onions

- Zucchini
- Yellow Squash
- Leeks
- Canned Green Beans

Fruit:

- Any berry
- Rhubarb
- Tomatoes in moderation
- Lemons
- Limes
- Avocado
- Coconut
- Figs
- Watermelon
- Cherries
- Pomegranate
- Papaya
- Raisins
- Plums
- Clementine
- Apple
- Guava

Dairy:

- Full Fat Milk
- Full Fat Greek Yogurt
- Mayonnaise
- Heavy Whipping Cream
- Sour Cream

Cheeses:

- Swiss
- String Cheese
- Parmesan
- Mozzarella
- Monterey Jack
- Goat Cheese
- Feta
- Cream Cheese
- Cottage Cheese
- Colby
- Cheddar
- Brie
- Blue

Meats:

- Beef
- Chicken
- Pork
- Turkey
- Tuna
- Salmon
- Cod
- Flounder
- Tilapia
- Shrimp
- Scallops
- Lobster

Spices:

- All herbs and spices

Dressings and Sauces:

- Lime Juice
- Lemon Juice
- Italian
- Ranch
- Blue Cheese
- Brown and Yellow Mustard
- Worcestershire Sauce
- Vinegar
- Soy Sauce
- Sugar-Free Syrup
- Sugar-Free Ketchup
- Low-Carb Salsa

Liquids:

- Protein Shakes
- Unsweetened Tea
- Coffee (can add heavy cream)
- Almond Milk
- Cashew Milk
- Coconut Milk

Oils and Fats:

- Sunflower Oil
- Sesame Oil
- Peanut Oil

- Olive Oil
- Mayonnaise
- Coconut Oil
- Bacon Fat
- Butter

Baking and Cooking:

- Cocoa Power
- Chia Seeds
- Flax Seeds
- Flax Meal
- Almond Meal/Flour
- Coconut Flakes
- Coconut Flour

Sweeteners:

- Xylitol
- Stevia Drops
- Erythritol

Evaluate Your Keto Diet Experience

With your meal plan and recipes ready to go and your mind ready for the diet, you begin. In the first week, things immediately start to get uncomfortable and your energy seems to have dropped to almost nonexistent levels. This shouldn't come as a surprise since this is normal for anyone and it is simply signs of your body being in a transition.

Common Side Effects

With any change to your diet, it is normal to have some side effects as your body begins to adapt to the new way you are eating. When doing a ketogenic diet, the body must switch the fuel source from glucose to fat stores. This can cause some of the following side effects:

Keto Flu

With your body used to only breaking down carbohydrates and using it for energy, it had built up numerous enzymes dedicated to this process. Because of the body's dependence on carbohydrates, it neglected the production of enzymes for dealing with fats. Then, your body is suddenly dealing with a lack of glucose and constant supply of fats, which triggers the body to start producing enzymes for using fat as fuel.

However, this would take time and not only one or two days. The first few weeks on a keto diet is challenging for some and easy for others. Your body is used to relying on glucose for energy, so it needs to switch to using ketones for fuel. This can result in brain fog but disappears when the body gets adapted. This adaptation takes about four weeks, but the side effects disappear sooner. Around the end of the first week, it is normal to feel some flu-like symptoms like cravings, insomnia, racing heart when lying down, fatigue, dizziness and brain fog. You can lessen these effects by gradually lowering your carb intake over a few weeks. If you decide to just right into a keto diet, just remember to get plenty of fluids and salts. This will keep you from feeling lousy.

This is called Keto Flu and is a natural transitional response of your body. This usually happens during the first week of your ketogenic diet. In this state, you will experience headaches, mental fogginess, dizziness and aggravation. These ailments are due to your electrolytes being eliminated in your body because ketones have a diuretic effect. To counteract this, you should drink plenty of water and increase the sodium in your body.

<u>Curing the Keto Flu</u>

The keto flu will vary with each person. Many find the symptoms are worst in the first week. Some find they linger for weeks on end. There are some tricks you can do to shorten your flu time:

- Eat more fats: This is a common method used to combat the keto flu. Your body needs energy. It isn't getting it from sugar and carbs, so it needs to get it from what you are eating. Eat lots of healthy fats like lard, tallow, ghee, olive oil and coconut oil. To stay in ketosis, you need to consume plenty of fats. Adding MCT oil can boost your ketone level. This will help your brain feel better.
- Eat more calories: It is easy to not eat enough when you begin a low carb diet. Many just cut out the carbs without increasing other food intakes. They get confused about what they can eat since they are used to eating bread, rice and pasta.
- Exercise: This might be the last thing you are thinking about right now. Studies show that exercise helps you to become more metabolically flexible. This means that your body can switch between carbs and ketones for energy easily. People that don't experience the keto flu for long are more metabolically flexible because they can switch between ketones and carbs.

Bad Breath

This is sometimes called keto breath. It can happen as you go into ketosis. Ketones get released into the breath, sweat and urine. Acetone is one form of a ketone that is released in the breath and can cause a metallic taste in the mouth. This is temporary and will disappear after a couple of weeks. If this becomes a problem, sugar-free breath fresheners or gum can help. You can increase your oral hygiene by using mouthwash and brushing your teeth more often.

Leg Cramps

Developing muscle cramps might be possible with the keto diet. These can sometimes be rather bothersome. The cause of cramps is a condition called hyponatremia. This happens when salt levels are too low. Stay hydrated and add salt to the diet.

Loss of Salts

There will be changes in your fluid balance in the first few weeks on the keto diet. This happens as the body uses up the stored sugars that in turn release water into the blood that gets flushed out through the urine. When fluids get passed out, salts in the body will become depleted. Keep yourself hydrated. Water is best, but coffee and tea are fine as long as they aren't extremely milky. Make sure you have plenty of salt, so you won't experience side effects like wooziness and headaches. You can add sea salt to your food and drink bone or vegetable bouillons and broths. Magnesium and potassium are important salts, too.

If you are eating natural, healthy foods like vegetables, dairy, fish, meat and nuts, you shouldn't have any problems getting the potassium and magnesium you need.

Bowel Habit Change

A keto diet can cause constipation. The body's gut bacteria need to adapt to be able to handle the different foods and the different amounts of food. Bowel habits usually improve in a couple of weeks. If they don't, make sure you are getting enough fiber. Drink lots of water and increase the amounts of seeds, nuts, legumes and fibrous vegetables.

Loss of Energy

The biggest misconception of the keto diet is the lack of glucose will deplete the body of its energy. Keeping steady energy is more challenging with a standard diet because it fluctuates with blood sugar.

Eating lower carbs doesn't prevent the sugar level rollercoaster. Once the body gets into ketosis, the body begins to draw energy from its fat stores. The liver begins to create the amount of glucose the body needs.

By cutting down on carbs, the body will find it easier to regulate energy and sugar level. You might notice a dip in energy while adapting to the diet; this should pass in a few weeks.

Poor Physical Performance

Due to low levels of blood sugar, your physical performance will drop. This is only for the short term and your body will eventually adapt to it. However, if you have to always be on top of your performance, it will be beneficial for you if you adopt either the Cyclic or Targeted Ketogenic Diet. These two approaches will provide you the energy for your physical activities and, at the same time, enable you to have a ketogenic diet.

Other than that, you may also experience cramps, constipation and heart palpitations. These are easily remedied by your proper hydration and by eating foods with good sources of micronutrients. There is nothing to be alarmed when you experience these effects. In fact, they tell you that your body is adjusting to a state of ketosis.

These side effects are normally temporary and can be remedied.

Signs that you've reached Ketosis
- Bad breath due to acetone, a ketone being expelled through your mouth or urine.
- Dry mouth and increased thirst due to ketones being diuretics.
- Increased urination

What to watch out for

It is important to keep track of your ketones to make sure that your body is responding to the diet and to prevent ketoacidosis. It is when the ketones in your body approach dangerous levels. Although it is easy to assume that ketones can reach high levels, this is simply not true and is, in fact, a rare occurrence.

It is still important to regularly keep track of your ketones. This can easily be done and no need for laboratory tests to be done. Ketone testing can easily be done through urine strips, breath ketone analyzers and blood ketone meter.

Keeping up Motivation

Beginning a new diet is exciting. You see all the transformation pictures online and you start to see how your body will change, also. Sticking to a keto diet until it becomes your lifestyle gets challenging. If you can stick to the keto diet for a few months, you will get the results of more energy, mental clarity and loss of body fat. Here are some techniques to help you:

1. Start small. It is tempting to go all in in the beginning. Your motivation will be high and we have a tendency to push ourselves to the limit. We think we have to cook all our meals at home instead of going out to eat. We

have to join a gym and work out for hours five days a week. This will cause the body to crash and burn and the result is stopping the diet completely. The answer to this is the pick a small change that is easy to commit to. If you want to change your whole diet, start by changing your breakfast. Don't go to the gym for hours every day just do 15 minutes two times a week. By starting small, it will be impossible not to do it. Create the habit first and then increase it once you have gained traction.

2. Eat the same things. The reason many people don't stick to a diet is that they are looking for a variety each day. If they get stressed out or their willpower is tested, they just go to a fast food restaurant. If they can learn to eat the same meals each day, it will reduce the likelihood of cheating since you already know what you are going to eat. Repeat the same three or four meal over and over. Try variety on the weekends.

3. Take some food with you. We might not always be around keto friendly food. It might be a family gathering or a party at work. The temptation is everywhere. The key here is controlling your environment. Pack a lunchbox or backpack full of keto-friendly snacks to take with you wherever you go. If you begin to feel tempted grab a handful and eat away. This might save you from cheating on your diet.

4. Make success rewarding. Most people know how to lose weight. Having a true reason to change is the answer, not more information. Use positive reinforcements to help. Set realistic weight loss goals for yourself like losing ten pounds in 30 days. Think of something that you have wanted to do for a long time like taking a trip someplace you've never been or spending the day at a spa. You can only do this if you reach your weight loss goal.

5. Never try to be perfect. Stay focused on the progress, not perfection. Be okay with grabbing a non-keto snack every now and then. Too many have

quit reaching for their goal because they think they have failed. We are all human. To err is human. The real failure here is just giving up.

Long-Term Tips

No matter how much you love the ketogenic diet, there are family reunions, parties and other events that can easily derail your best-laid plans. Holidays and birthdays can be particularly difficult, as you are surrounded by sweet and savory dishes that bring back fond memories. Being surrounded by relatives and friends who lovingly prepared all of the food can make resisting even more difficult. Having to prepare food separately from what you feed your family can be difficult. Additionally, you are probably finding that the ketogenic diet takes a lot of commitment. Food preparation, storage and grocery shopping can take vastly larger amounts of time than before. Plus, it costs more than eating a high-carb diet. Here are some tips to help you stay on the ketogenic diet long-term.

Plan ahead

Planning your meals in advance is a strategic way to manage a busy schedule while sticking to a healthy eating plan. Prepare your grocery list before you go to the store so that you don't forget anything that you need. Having to make an extra grocery trip during the week can easily cost you an hour or two.

Make sure that you always have keto-friendly foods on you. Invest in some food containers that you can easily put in your bag and take with you places. Keep them filled with things like nuts, vegetable sticks, yogurt dip and sliced avocados. At a sports game, in a meeting, out on a long shopping excursion, or anytime that you have to be away from home for more than a few hours, you can pop the containers out and recharge on ketogenic foods.

One challenge of the ketogenic diet is that many foods have to be eaten immediately after being prepared. The thought of eating scrambled eggs that have been in the refrigerator for a couple of days is less than appetizing. Look for recipes that can be prepared in advance and eaten throughout the week. Examples include curries, soups and casseroles. Take one day each week to prepare some dishes that can be refrigerated and eaten throughout the week. This will save you a lot of time and enable you to stay on track, even on your busiest days.

Know what local restaurants have keto-friendly options on their menus so that when you do go out to eat, you already know what you can order without derailing your diet. Just because something isn't labeled keto-friendly doesn't mean that it isn't. An omelet with cheese is probably fine, as long as you don't add hash browns or anything else on the side. If you are at a restaurant that doesn't have anything that appears to be keto-friendly, ask for something to be specially prepared, based on the ingredients that appear in the other foods on the menu. For example, if there are choices that contain avocados, cucumbers and oil and vinegar dressing, you can request that those ingredients be made into a salad.\

Take advantage of grocery delivery

Grocery shopping can be a time-consuming hassle, but nowadays, many stores offer grocery delivery. You select online what you want and when you want it to be delivered, then pay online via credit or debit card. This can shave hours every week off of the time you spend on maintaining your keto diet.

Keep in mind that grocery delivery usually carries a fee and may be more expensive than going to the store, so make sure that you are aware of the cost. If you live in a large city, there may be several different stores that offer grocery delivery that you can check out.

Let others know of your diet

Before going out with friends or going to visit relatives, let them know that you are on the ketogenic diet. Inform them that you don't expect them to prepare any special food for you but that there are many foods that you will not be able to eat. Try to select restaurants that you know have keto-friendly options so that you and your friends can enjoy eating whatever you prefer. And who knows? You may find that others want to join you on the ketogenic diet!

Make friends with others who are on the ketogenic diet

Joining a group of people who are already on the ketogenic diet can be a great way to achieve accountability with people who are working towards the same goals. People who have already been where you are can give you practical advice about how they dealt with the side effects of adjusting to the diet and a state of ketosis, as well as how to handle things like the holidays and those worried emails from your parents about the supposed dangers of going keto. They can also give you pointers about things like saving money on groceries and cooking keto meals separately from what your family normally eats.

While you should avoid preaching to your friends about going keto, some may see how much the diet has benefited you and want to join in. You can hook them up with your buddies who are already on the ketogenic diet and work together as accountability partners.

Exercise regularly

The benefits of exercise are so immense that it is a wonder that doctors don't prescribe it instead of medication. It boosts immunity, improves blood flow and circulation, elevates mood, increases metabolism, burns off the stress hormones that can accumulate after traumatic events or as part of a hectic daily life, burns calories, purges blood sugar, relieves constipation, reduces insulin, the list goes on and on. One reason nutritionists may be against the ketogenic diet is that it doesn't necessarily incorporate exercise.

Commonly, people get onto the ketogenic diet as a shortcut to losing weight instead of as part of a healthy lifestyle, which has to include exercise. If you go onto the ketogenic diet, it needs to be because you want to improve your health, not just because you want to lose weight. Losing weight is a side effect of increased health and wellness. You need to exercise for at least thirty minutes four times a week.

Going for a brisk walk in the evening or for a morning jog is a great way to get started with exercise. Taking the stairs instead of the elevator and parking further away from the store instead of fighting for a front-row parking spot are easy ways to incorporate exercise into your daily life. You may want to join a gym or buy in-home exercise equipment, but you don't have to. Most people who buy gym membership or exercise equipment never use it unless they were already exercising regularly beforehand.

The best way to make exercise a meaningful and regular part of your life is to make it enjoyable. Put on some music and listen to your favorite songs while you are running on the treadmill. Go for a walk with your family or a friend. You will soon find that you feel so much better, both physically and emotionally, that you will want to continue exercising as much as possible.

Plan keto nights with friends

Your friends and/or family don't understand the ketogenic diet and they frequently discourage you from following it. Your mom repeatedly sends you emails with articles about how dangerous the ketogenic diet is and your best friend keeps tempting you with your favorite carb-rich foods to try to get you to start eating "normally" again. They have no idea why you would spend so much time preparing high-fat meals at home. So show them!

Plan keto nights in which you prepare keto-friendly foods for your friends and family to try. Have all of the ingredients out and enlist their help to prepare the meal. They might find themselves pleasantly surprised at how appetizing the ketogenic diet really is and some might even decide to join you!

Drink lots of water

Because the water-rich foods that you probably once enjoyed, like mangoes and apples, are no longer staples in your diet, you are consuming significantly less water than before. Additionally, when you are first starting out on the ketogenic diet, your kidneys will have to work harder to process all of the fat you are consuming along with the glucose and glycogen stores that your body is burning through. You will have to be intentional about drinking a lot of water. You will probably need to drink one ounce for every pound of body weight. If you are 160 pounds, you will probably need 160 ounces of water per day.

Practice intermittent fasting

Intermittent fasting is the practice of fasting for between 16 and 48 hours at a time for the purpose of gaining health benefits. Intermittent fasting has numerous health benefits. It turns on your body's fat burning processes, improves mental clarity and gets you into a state of ketosis.

You naturally are going into a fasting state at night when you sleep, because you aren't eating. Intermittent fasting extends this state throughout the day. Some experts prescribe fasts as a prelude to beginning the ketogenic diet and others advise fasts as a way to get the most benefits out of it. This is actually much easier than you may think because the ketogenic diet leads to significantly less hunger. When fasting, make sure that you consume plenty of fluids. You may want to supplement with things like coconut oil and butter to help induce ketosis.

Decrease your stress levels

Many of us live hectic, stressful lives. We are busy from the time we wake up until we go to sleep and increasing demands are constantly placed on us. You may find that you are constantly stressed to please your boss at work, care for your children and/or aging parents, maintain your home, keep up with finances, the list goes on and on. Our use of smartphones keeps us constantly connected, which can easily mean that the boss expects us to be readily available to answer emails and phone calls after hours. With today's tough economy, you may find that you are working a lot of extra hours or even two jobs (or more!) to try to stay afloat financially. Just let it be said that stress is an epidemic and you are probably not immune to it.

The effects of stress can be disastrous for anyone's health. In response to stress, the body releases cortisol and adrenaline and induces a "fight or flight" response. Many people actually live in a perpetual fight-or-flight state and are unable to shut their minds down, even to be able to sleep at night. The cortisol causes fat to build up in the abdominal area, which is the most harmful place for fat to accumulate. Stress also causes blood pressure to rise and increases the risk of other heart diseases. It easily makes people irritable, causing harmful effects on their relationships. Mood disorders, like depression and anxiety, can develop. Chronic stress can also lead to autoimmune problems, digestive issues, insomnia, skin problems like eczema and acne, infertility and cognitive issues. It can also inhibit a state of ketosis because stress hormones actually raise blood sugar and insulin and drive down ketone production. Needless to say, reducing stress is an important step in maintaining a healthy lifestyle.

Think about what you can reasonably do to decrease the stress in your life. You may need to take major steps, like considering a job change or lowering your hours at work. You may need to make other small changes, like reducing your financial obligations or turning off your smartphone at certain hours. Many people find that working with a counselor to help them deal with the toxic effects of stress and identify its causes is very beneficial in improving their quality of life.

You may be going through a particularly stressful or even traumatic period in your life. If that is the case, maintaining a state of ketosis may not be a reasonable goal. Instead, aim to eat a low-carb, high-fat diet, exercise regularly and seek out support from family, friends and possibly a professional.

Monitor your health

Because the ketogenic diet induces so many chemical changes in your body's metabolism, you need to keep tabs on different markers of health. You can easily buy ketone-testing strips that measure your ketone production through breath, blood, or urine. The ketogenic diet tends to reduce the electrolytes in your body, so you may want to get a tool that measures electrolytes in order to ensure you have an adequate amount. Because the goal of the ketogenic diet is ultimately to suppress the use of glucose for energy by inducing ketosis, you may want to get some tools for testing your blood sugar and insulin levels. These tools are easily available, as they are frequently used by diabetics as part of their daily regimens.

There are easy ways to monitor whether or not you are dehydrated. If your urine is yellow, cloudy and/or has a strong odor, you are probably dehydrated and need to drink a lot of water. This can also mean that you are drinking enough fluids but not enough water, so cut back on things like milk, coffee and tea and replace them with water. Another dehydration test is to pinch your arm. If the skin immediately snaps back into place, you are fine. If it sags or takes a moment to return to its original position, then you are dehydrated.

If implemented correctly, the ketogenic diet can become a lifelong lifestyle of health and wellness that will improve your wellbeing for years to come.

Mistakes to Avoid

Now let's look at the top mistakes Keto Dieters make and strategies to overcome them. It is helpful to keep them in mind even after you are successfully leading a Keto Lifestyle.

Mistake 1: Not Knowing your Macro Proportions

Ketosis is a reversible phenomenon. So long as you are using fat as your primary food and burning ketones for energy you will be able to control your weight and blood sugar levels. As soon you switch back to carbs, eat too much of proteins or reduce the proportion of fat in your diet, the body goes back to burning sugar for energy.

That's why maintaining an optimum proportion of Fats, Proteins and Carbs in your diet is so important for a Ketogenic Diet. Majority of the people falter in keeping this balance of proportion in a sustainable way over a long period of time.

So what is the Optimum Proportion?

Again, the answer to this question is more nuanced than you would like to hear. In short, the answer is, Know Your Own Body. Please find the recommended ranges below, but you will have to work with your body to determine the optimum amounts suitable to keep you in Ketosis.

In terms of percentage ratio the following proportions are recommended:

- Fat 60-75%
- Protein 15-30%
- Carbs 5-10%

Broadly the proportion depends on the following factors:

- Your Body Mass Index
- Your Age
- Your Percentage Body Fat
- Your Activity Level

If you are just starting on your Keto Diet, it's best to restrict your carb intake to 20-30 grams per day (remember 1 big orange = 1 pint of beer = 20 grams carb). For a majority of people, carb intake range can be increased to 20-50 grams per day once you have achieved the desired weight loss and are in the weight maintenance phase. There are a number of Keto Calculator Apps you can find that will help you in calculating your exact macro proportions.

Mistake 2: Scale Watching

You need to accept the fact that being on a Keto Diet is a lifestyle change and not a crash diet. You will get there, keep calm and carry on!

It's natural for you to want to weigh yourself regularly to check progress when on a diet, but this is actually not a very accurate way to measure results. You need to realize that weight is just a number and is neither a very meaningful or accurate measure of how you are progressing nor an indicator of fat loss or physical fitness. Just remember that apart from your water weight that can fluctuate several pounds in a short span, the scale is a snapshot of what happened two weeks back.

What is the difference between your friend who weighs 300 lb. and an athlete who weighs the same? They do weigh the same but is their body composition the same?

It is important to understand that losing fat and weight are two different things. As we lose body fat and gain muscle mass especially for someone who has recently begun exercising, the scale would continue to show the same weight. Indicators that you are on track to losing weight even if the scale doesn't budge:

- Your tape measurements show a shrinking waistline.
- Your clothes are getting looser, you look slimmer and people around you notice the difference.
- You have lots of energy and want to exercise after living a sedentary lifestyle for years.
- Your health markers are improving.
- Your Body Mass Index (BMI) dips.
- Your mental focus improves, you don't experience afternoon slumps anymore.

Measure your Ketones

Measuring ketones is a good way to know that your body is in Ketosis and is burning the stored fat. There are a number of ways to measure ketones produced in your liver as your body goes through ketosis. These include urine test kits, blood test kits, breathalyzers and good old-fashioned observation techniques. Depending on your budget and interest, measuring ketones can be a good way to monitor results during ketogenic diet.

Mistake 3: Sugar Addiction

Sugar is the biggest hindrance to leading a healthy lifestyle. Removing sugar completely from your diet is absolutely necessary for a successful transition to Ketogenic Diet lifestyle. In fact, a gradual removal of this single substance from your diet alone will make you healthier than the majority of people. If you want to take one lesson from this book it is to completely remove sugar from your life.

The average per capita sugar consumption in America has risen to 153 grams per day from 9 grams per day back in 1822. Our bodies have got so used to sugar that in reality, it is difficult to get through a day without consuming sugar in some form. Being so readily available and ingrained in our lifestyle makes it all the more difficult to give up sweet foods. Check out the Resources section of the book for 56 different names of sugar used by the processed food industry to hide the amounts of added sugar in your food.

So what is Sugar? Sugar is simply Glucose + Fructose (The Sweet Part). It has:

- No healthy fats
- No protein
- No vitamins
- No enzymes

How Sugar makes us Eat More - Sugar triggers a chain reaction where high levels of sugar in the bloodstream results in increased insulin levels. This insulin, in turn, makes it difficult for the brain to receive the satiety signal. As a result, the brain is fooled to believe that the body is still hungry leading to excessive food consumption and weight gain.

How to Overcome Sugar Cravings:

• Reduce your Carb Intake: A high carb diet causes blood sugar to rise, which in turn signals the body to release insulin. You need to increase your consumption of protein and good fat to overcome this. Proteins are made up of amino acids, which are important for balancing hormones and sugar cravings. Healthy fats are a source of energy for our body and help reduce hunger pangs and provide satiety.

• Plan Your Meals in Advance: Hunger is not the best time to make rational decisions on what is best to eat. Planning ahead to include nutrient-rich food in your diet will help curb hunger swings and sugar cravings.

• L-Glutamine Dr. Julia Ross in her book "The Mood Curse" suggests that intense sugar cravings are due to stress, poor diet and deficiency of amino acids (to the extent that diet alone may not be able to correct it). She suggests a short-term supplementation of amino acid L- Glutamine.

• Check your Pantry: Keep sugary foods out of sight as much as possible.

• Watch Out for the Hidden Sugar: Low fat, sugar-free and diet foods contain added sugar or synthetic sweeteners in order to enhance the taste of the food and palatability. Get into the habit of going through the labeling for savory foods, juices, sauces, salad dressings and condiments. You will be surprised how many of them contain sugar.

• Avoid Artificial Sweeteners: Replacing sugar with a sugar substitute in the belief that it will reduce calorie intake and help in weight loss is a myth. Recent studies have shown that on the contrary artificial sweeteners maintain the cravings for sweet food and increase appetite. Our body increases insulin secretion in anticipation that sugar will appear in the bloodstream. When the body doesn't receive the sugar, insulin uses the existing sugar in the bloodstream for energy. As a result, blood sugar levels drop and hunger increases leading to uncontrolled binging.

Mistake 4: Electrolyte Imbalance

Electrolytes are salts that flow in your bloodstream and carry an electric charge. They are essential for the cells in our body to function properly, whether it is to regulate blood pressure, help with muscle contraction or nervous system functions.

It is a well-known fact that on a Keto Diet the initial transition phase results in significant water loss. With the water are lost essential minerals like sodium and potassium, which triggers an electrolyte imbalance.

You will need about three times more electrolytes when on a Keto Diet as compared to a normal diet. Signs that you have an Electrolyte Imbalance:

- You are restless, have muscle aches, spasms and joint pains
- You have heart palpitations and find it difficult to sleep.
- You experience dizziness and fatigue I

Important Electrolytes Include:

<u>Sodium</u>

Responsible for maintaining fluid balance in our bodies, helps in muscle contraction and nerve signaling.

Sources of Sodium: Table Salt and Himalayan Pink Salt.

Magnesium:

One of the most under-appreciated minerals, Magnesium helps in maintaining a stable heart rate, bone building, the creation of DNA and RNA and normal nerve and muscle functions.

Sources of Magnesium: Almond, Salmon, Spices and Leafy Vegetables.

Potassium:

It aids muscle contraction, regulates heart contractions and keeps blood pressure stable. An imbalance of sodium and potassium is caused when we consume sodium-loaded processed foods and skip vegetables rich in potassium. This could lead to hypertension, heart attack and stroke.
Sources of Potassium: Avocado, Nuts and Dark Leafy Vegetables.

Calcium:

In addition to helping with the formation and maintenance of bones and teeth, calcium helps with cell division, cell clotting and transmission of nerve impulses.

Sources of Calcium: Almonds, Cheese and Broccoli.

Healthy individuals who are not working out extensively get their daily intake of electrolytes from the food they eat.

However, if you are sick, out on a very hot day or on a low carb diet, your electrolyte requirement spikes up.

Mistake 5: Fat Phobia

For years we have been told that eating fat will make you fat. Some of the most popular diets in the world are based on this premise. It is this social conditioning that leads us to subconsciously make choices that are low in fat.

As a result sugar and grains have been the primary source of the calories for most of us. Once you remove these two from your diet you will need to replace them with another energy source. If you don't you will feel hungry, tired and low all the time and will eventually switch back to carbs.

It is important to understand that there are two sources of energy – glucose and ketones. When on a low carb diet, sufficient intake of fat (60-75 % of total intake) leads us into ketosis and our body uses ketones for energy. However, if our body does not get into ketosis, it will look out for glucose for energy. It will either get it from carbohydrates or from protein (through Gluconeogenesis).

Keto Diet advocates a mix of saturated fats, omega 3s and monounsaturated fats.

Different types of Fat Present in our Food:

Saturated Fat (SFA):

They are stable fats, with long shelf life and suitable for high flame cooking. They help to keep in check your bone density, immune system and testosterone levels. Contrary to popular belief their consumption does not adversely affect the heart.

Sources of SFA: Meat, Egg, Butter, Ghee, Lard, Coconut Oil are good sources of Saturated Fat.

Monounsaturated Fat (MUFA):

They are liquid at room temperature and best for cold use for salads or after cooking. Good for the heart, they are now a popular choice of fat.

Sources of MUFA: Avocado, Olives and Nuts (especially macadamia).

Polyunsaturated Fat (PUFA):

This type of fats can be primarily divided into the naturally occurring Omega 3s and the industrially processed Omega 6 fats. PUFAs are unstable and fragile and not suitable for cooking. When heated, they react with oxygen to form harmful compounds called free radicals, which in turn raise our risk of heart diseases and cancer. Omega 3 consumption is good for our body but most of the PUFA cooking oil is high in omega 6, which is harmful.

The ideal ratio of Omega 6 to Omega 3 fats is 1: 1. However, in reality, the ratio is way higher than this, ranging from 10: 1 to 20: 1 on an average, so not only do we have a problem of excess Polyunsaturated fat, we also have a much higher proportion of omega 6 fats and deficiency of omega 3s.

Sources of healthy Omega 3s: Wild Salmon, Walnut, Fermented Cod Liver Oil, Macadamia Nuts and Grass-Fed Meat.

Trans Fat:

This is considered the worst form of fat and should be avoided. Trans fat is unsaturated fats primarily found in processed foods where through industrial process hydrogen is added to liquid vegetable oil to cause the fat to become solid at room temperature. This partially hydrogenated oil helps to increase the shelf life of processed food. It is linked to heart diseases and has an adverse effect on cholesterol levels.

Stay clear of products whose product label mentions words like "trans fat", "hydrogenated". It is worth noting that in the United States if per serving of any product anything lower than 0.5 grams then it can be labeled as 0 grams of trans fat. These hidden trans fats quickly add up if you consume multiple servings.

High-Fat Foods to Include in Your Diet:

- Avocados: Avocado, unlike most fruit, is loaded with monounsaturated fat oleic acid. This is the main fatty acid in olive oil and linked with various health benefits. It is a great source of potassium and fiber and helps lower triglyceride.
- Cheese: It is made from the milk of grass-fed animals is a good source of nutrients as it is high in saturated fats and omega 3-s, protein and amino acids
- Whole Eggs: Eggs are one of the most nutrient-dense foods and are loaded with vitamins and minerals.
- Fatty cuts of Meats and Fish: Include fatty cuts of grass-fed animals. Avoid chicken breasts or lean meat where the fat has been removed. Include fish like Salmon, Sardine, Mackerel and Trout in the meal plans. If you cannot eat fish then it is worth considering a supplement like Cod fish liver oil, which contains Omega 3-s and Vitamin D.

- Nuts: Nuts are loaded with Protein, Vitamin E and Magnesium in addition to healthy fats and are a great option to add to a meal when consumed in moderation. Almonds, Walnuts and Macadamia nuts are some of the healthy choices.
- Chia seeds: They are high in Omega 3 fatty acids and fiber. They can be a useful addition to your diet.
- Extra Virgin Olive Oil: Rich in vitamin E & K and loaded with antioxidants, extra virgin Olive oil is an excellent choice. The antioxidants in the oil help improve cardiovascular health, lower blood pressure, fight inflammation and protect LDL particles from oxidation in the blood.
- Coconut Oil: It contains 90% saturated fatty acids making it the richest source of saturated fat.
- Butter and Ghee (clarified butter): Butter has been demonized for long but Grass Fed butter is good for you. In addition to Vitamin A, E and K2 it contains Conjugated Linoleic Acid (CLA) and Butyrate. CLA helps in lowering fat percentage and Butyrate improves the gut and fights inflammation.
- Lard, Tallow and Bacon Fat from naturally raised animals are a great option for cooking and are high in healthy saturated and monounsaturated fats

Mistake 6: Carb-Loaded

So much has already been discussed about carbs. But I would like to reiterate that you should become aware of your carb tolerance. An athlete will probably have a greater carb tolerance than someone with a sedentary lifestyle. On the safer side, your carbs intake should not go beyond 20 grams max when you start your Keto Diet.

Getting rid of carbs may work in the short term, but there always comes a time when all of us start to crave for the starchy stuff. The temptation of having just that one small slice of bread can be overwhelming.

Let me warn you again though, Ketosis is a reversible state and can be broken very easily by just having that one small piece. Not only that, once you start eating that one piece, insulin level in your blood starts to rise which will play all kinds of havoc with you. Let me show you how a high carb diet affects us physiologically.

Why "Eat less and Exercise more" is Not a Solution: The conventional weight loss wisdom from the diet industry is 'Eat less and Exercise more'. This advice, derived from the calorie in calorie out (CICO) theory, falls flat in the world of complex human physiology. CICO completely ignores the inner workings of a human body and has led to lots of people abandoning their weight loss quest.

People who propagate CICO believe that Calorie IN = Calorie OUT + Stored Fat. So the amount of fat stored in the body depends upon the number of calories we consume minus the calories expended in bodily functions and exercise. Nothing can be far from the truth!

The human body has no way of measuring calories but has its own way of regulating fat. Insulin is the hormone that controls how much energy we expend and how much is stored as fat.

When we eat, the insulin goes up and the body starts storing fat. And eating equal calories of carb will raise insulin level more that eating equal calories of fat. That's why in human physiology; a calorie is not a calorie. As we stop eating, the insulin levels drop and the body stops storing fat. As the fasting continues body starts burning the stored fat.

That's why conventional (High Carb Low Fat) diets fail. Because of high insulin levels in carb-based diets, fat is being continuously stored. So even if you are eating lesser calories overall, insulin levels will remain high because of carb consumption and fat storage will continue. Ironically, weight gain continues and with increased appetite.

In a Low Carb High Fat (LCHF) diet, however, the insulin levels are lower. So when you consume equal calories of fat based food, a part of your energy needs will be met with the stored body fat. So using an LCHF diet for fat loss is more effective as your appetite is decreasing with a steady decline in body fat.

Mistake 7: Excessive Drinking

Keto Diet does not mean the end of your social life. Sure hit the bars, but you have to do so responsibly. Please remember if it tastes sweet, it's probably sugary and should be avoided.

You will have to keep a check on what you drink and how much you drink. Beer and wine should be especially avoided as they contain a lot of carbs and sugar. When you drink, your body will metabolize it on priority before other sources of energy, as it cannot store alcohol. This means that although alcohol consumption will not completely throw you out of ketosis it will for sure prolong the timeline for your goals as when the body is burning alcohol for energy it is unable to metabolize the stored fat.

Remember to drink plenty of water in between your drinks. Keto lowers your alcohol tolerance level so keep sufficient gap between drinks.

Mistake 8: Importance of Proteins

Like many of us do you also have the notion that Ketogenic Diet is all about keeping your carbs low and increasing your fat intake?

For a lot of people just keeping low on carbs, helps in weight loss. However, some people are more metabolically resistant than others and despite keeping their carb levels below 20 grams per day continue to gain weight. It is in such cases worth looking at your protein intake.

We give little attention to how much protein we need to consume in order to stay in ketosis. Our body cannot make protein on its own and as such protein is an important macronutrient without which your body wouldn't be able to carry out the necessary tissue building and repair functions.

What is Gluconeogenesis?

It is worth understanding the process of gluconeogenesis here. It is a metabolic process by which our body produces glucose from non-carbohydrate sources – amino acids in the protein being one of them.

Gluconeogenesis is an essential process without which we probably cannot survive for long, especially if we need to go without food, as our body needs a constant and steady flow of glucose to keep the brain and red blood cells functioning.

When we consume more protein than our body needs the excess is turned into glucose. This glucose is over and above the minimum requirement of the body and results in weight gain.

Optimum Protein Intake:

There are various theories on how you can calculate the ideal protein intake taking your weight in pounds and then multiply it by 0.6 and 1.0. This will then give you the ideal range for your protein intake in grams.

An easier way is to pick a level of protein and while still keeping carbs below 20 grams monitor how you are doing for that quantity of protein intake. If you continue to struggle, keep shifting your intake downwards until you hit the sweet spot.

It is worth noting that when you are experimenting to find your ideal level of protein intake you must keep your carbs low and have adequate monounsaturated and saturated fats to give you the much-needed satiety.

If you are struggling with weight loss due to being more sensitive to proteins, try and avoid leaner cuts of meat like chicken breast as that would elevate your blood sugar levels and make you gain weight just by having too much protein than your body needs. On the other side, cuts of meats with saturated fat will automatically lower your protein intake and help in weight loss.

Mistake 9: Falling for Fake Products

Wouldn't it be great if we could eat bread, pasta and chocolate and still lose weight rapidly without hunger or all the complicated diseases associated with sugar?

There are plenty of shady businesses that promise the impossible. An excellent example is low carb pasta from Dreamfields that tastes like any regular pasta. They are even made from regular starchy wheat, but the manufacturer still claims that our body does not absorb the carbs as their pasta is protected from some "patent pending process".

The problem is that their claims are completely bogus and raises blood sugar like any regular pasta. Based on several types of research it was proved that their pasta behaved like regular pasta and Dreamfields had to pay a settlement fine of $ 8 million because they had lied; however, by then they had sold their fake low carb pasta for 10 years.

There are many similar examples of fake products. Carbzone is a company that claims to sell low carb products. They claim their tortilla made from whole wheat is low carb; however, on testing it showed to contain 3 times as many carbs as stated on the label. Even low carb chocolate cookies from the Atkins Company often contain sugar alcohol like Maltitol, which the maker pretends to not raise blood sugar. However, this claim has no merit and about half of it does end up raising blood sugar. The manufactures omit sugar alcohols from the net carb count so that they can market it as low carb.

In short, do not fall for fake products. If it tastes like bread, pasta or chocolate then the reality is that it is bread, pasta and chocolate.

Lifestyle Problems

Now, let's look at the lifestyle challenges that some followers may face. We will also look at the best ways that these can be addressed.

Keto on a Budget

Some people worry about following Ketogenic Diet on a budget. But actually, once you start, you'll find that your monthly spend on food will actually go down. The reasons for the same are mentioned below:
1. You will buy fresh base ingredients instead of processed ingredients
2. Once you hit ketosis, you will observe that satiety comes much earlier and you will eat less. This is another sign that you are in the state of Ketosis.

Farmer's market is a great place to shop for fresh ingredients while on Keto. You will find pocket-friendly bargains

there while supporting the local community. Moreover, you will learn more about your food by being in direct touch with the producers.

Eating Out

Eating in a restaurant can seem daunting when you first start following a ketogenic diet. Actually, it doesn't need to be difficult if you follow a few simple rules.

Try to stick to meat, dairy, or vegetable dishes that don't come with rice, pasta, or bread. Things like steak with salad are a good choice, as are salads on their own with cheese or meat added. Other good choices when eating out can be fish or seafood with non-starchy vegetables.

Just be careful to have them with olive oil rather than dressings, which can be high in sugar. Also remember that it is up to you if you want to customize your order and ask for things like sauces to be left out, so don't be afraid to ask! It also is worth checking with the restaurants if they have Keto/ Paleo/ LCHF friendly dishes.

Eating with Friends and Family

Friends and family may not understand Ketogenic Diet and may want you to eat whatever they are eating, especially if you have done so in the past. At the end of the day, you may not be able to explain the principles of Ketogenic Diet to them in a way that changes their minds, but just remember that it is up to you to choose what to eat. They may just be convinced when they see your weight loss and renewed energy levels!

Conclusion

The keto diet can be hard to maintain which is why you should try to get into it slowly. The first step is to slowly transition yourself into it instead of just pushing your body to the limit. So, don't abandon all the food that you used to eat, instead cut them out of your diet slowly.

The second step is to jump right into it and wait for the benefits to start showing. Now, it might happen that the diet isn't working for you, but you shouldn't worry about that. Our bodies are different which is why not all diets can work for everyone. You should consult your doctor if you are not losing any weight even after following the diet for a long time.

Lastly, remember to stay motivated and tell yourself why you're doing this. It can be hard to cut out all the carbs from your life, but you can always use some simple techniques to keep yourself motived. You should take pictures of yourself after every few months and notice the progress you are making, this will help you to stay on track.

Finally, if you enjoyed this book, then I'd like to ask you for a favor, would you be kind enough to leave a review for this book on Amazon? It'd be greatly appreciated!

Thank you and good luck!

Preview Of Intermittent fasting:
Beginners Guide To Weight Loss For Men And Women With Intermittent Fasting

Do you want a diet that will help you lose weight and improve your overall health? Do you want a diet that doesn't prescribe calorie counting? It does sound quite wonderful if you can achieve your weight loss and health goals without counting calories, doesn't it? If your answer is yes, then you are in for a pleasant surprise! Intermittent Fasting is the diet that you have been looking for. Fasting is not a new concept and has been around for a long time. Intermittent Fasting is a simple variation of fasting and is very helpful. This dieting protocol alternates between periods of fasting and eating.

In this book, you will learn about the basics of Intermittent Fasting, the changes that take place in your body, the benefits it offers, different methods of Intermittent Fasting, tips to exercise, common FAQs and much more. Intermittent Fasting is quite simple. You merely need to make a couple of changes to your eating habits and you are good to go.

If you are fascinated by this diet and want to learn more about it, then let us start right now!

Chapter One:
History of Intermittent Fasting

Unlike other forms of conventional dieting, the concept of fasting is quite unambiguous and easy to understand. Did you know that most of us tend to unconsciously follow the protocols of Intermittent Fasting? Do you ever skip having breakfast or dinner? If you do, then you are following an Intermittent Fasting protocol. You will learn about the different methods of Intermittent Fasting in the coming chapters.

Our hunter and gatherer caveman ancestors had to seek food in nature. So, they were often on a fast until they found some nourishment. Then agriculture was introduced, and it led to the formation of human civilization. Whenever there was food scarcity or whenever the seasons changed, fasting was the norm. They used to maintain stocks of grain and meat in cities and castles for harsh winters. Before the introduction of agriculture, shortage of rainfall meant a spell of famine and people used to fast to make their food supplies last longer. Enough rain was quintessential to meet the grain requirement.

Along with civilizations, there came religions. Religions grew when people were living in close quarters and shared similar beliefs. Most of the religions prescribe fasting. Hinduism refers to fasting as Vaasa, and Hindus observe it during festivals or other auspicious days. Fasting is also considered to be a form of penance. Islam prescribes fasting during the holy month of Ramzan. A similar practice is present in Judaism and is known as Yom Kippur. There's a period of fasting before Easter in the Catholic faith.

Technology and innovations play a vital role in the evolution of humans. Industrialization revolutionized the food industry. Mass production of food products meant that the markets were constantly flooded with food products. Apart from this, the way humans view and consume food has also undergone a major change. The human body didn't get a chance to sufficiently adapt itself to the rampant changes brought about by industrialization and agriculture. All this meant that a host of health problems soon followed. Intermittent Fasting is quite an old practice. Even though it is an old practice, humans have just begun to understand and truly appreciate the various benefits this diet offers. Whenever you fast, you give your body a chance to cleanse itself - not just cleanse but even repair and regenerate itself from within.

Essentially, while fasting your body gets to burn out all the excess fat it has stored. Human beings have evolved in such a manner that we can fast without any health risks and that is normal. Body fat is the reserve of food that the body has stashed away for a rainy day. If you don't consume food, your body will simply reach into this reserve to provide you with energy. There needs to be balance in everything you do. There's a yin and a yang. The same rule applies to eating and fasting as well. Fasting is the flip side of eating. If you aren't eating, then you are fasting. When you eat something, this leads to an accumulation of food energy that isn't going to be made use of immediately. A portion of this is stored away. A hormone known as insulin is responsible for storing the food energy. When you eat something, there is a spike in the level of insulin. This facilitates the storage of energy in two different ways. Sugars are linked into long chains and this is known as glycogen. The rest is stored in the liver. When the space available has been maxed out, the liver starts turning the rest into fat. Some of this fat so created is stored in the liver and the rest is stored in the form of fat cells in the rest of your body. There isn't a limit on fat creation. So, there are two forms of energy stores in our bodies. One is easily accessible and has a limited storage space (glycogen), and the other is the harder to reach energy without a limit on storage (body fat).

This process is essentially reversed when you don't eat, that is during fasting. There will be a reduction in the level of insulin and this enables your body to reach into its storage of fat cells and burn this to provide energy. The most easily attainable source of energy for your body is glycogen. This is broken down into molecules of glucose that sustains your body. This can provide sufficient energy for your body to function for 24 hours or longer. After this, your body will reach into its fat reserves to generate energy. Your body will do this only while feeding or fasting. Either your body will be storing energy, or it will be burning energy. Only either of these processes can take place at any given time. If there is a balance between eating and fasting, then there will not be any weight gain. Over a period of time, you will start gaining weight if you haven't given your body sufficient time to burn all the food it has stored. To restore balance, you will need to give your body sufficient time to burn the food energy. This can be accomplished by fasting. This is how our bodies are designed. Intermittent Fasting helps to restore this much-needed balance.

Circadian Rhythm and Intermittent Fasting

Human beings, like other organisms, have a biological circadian clock that ensures that the physiological processes in the body are performed at the right time. The circadian rhythm is on all day long and it affects the biology and the behavior of humans. Any disruption in this rhythm has a negative effect on the metabolism and it can cause several metabolic dysfunctions like obesity, diabetes and a host of cardiovascular diseases. The primary factor that affects the circadian rhythm is the signal to eat. It is responsible for metabolic, physiological and behavioral pathways in the body. All these pathways are responsible for making sure that your body performs optimally. Apart from this, they also ensure that your body is healthy. You can use behavioral intervention to regulate the body's circadian rhythm. Yes, you guessed it right! Intermittent Fasting is a means of behavioral intervention that will streamline the circadian rhythm. This in turn leads to better gene expression and improvement in your body's health and metabolism.

Gut Microbiome and Intermittent Fasting

The gastrointestinal tract regulates multiple processes within your body. In other words, your gut helps regulate different physiological and biochemical functions in your body. For instance, the metabolic reaction to glucose and the blood flow are higher during the day than at night. Even a small fluctuation in the circadian rhythm can impair your metabolism and increases the risk of several chronic diseases. The microbiome present in the gut is usually referred to as the second brain. It is known as the second brain because of the influence it has over your metabolism and physiology. Intermittent Fasting has a positive impact on the gut microbiome. It makes the gut less permeable, reduces the chances of systemic inflammation and improves overall energy balance.

Lifestyle Behavior and Intermittent Fasting

Intermittent Fasting helps change different health-related behaviors like calorie consumption, energy expenditure and your sleep cycle. Therefore, it is not a surprise that these are the three primary functions that help fight the most significant health concern that plagues the human community, obesity. You will learn more about the different benefits it offers in the coming chapters.

Chapter Two:
Different Methods of Fasting

Intermittent Fasting is a varied and a dynamic diet that offers multiple health benefits. There are different methods of Intermittent Fasting that you can follow, and you need to select one that will meet your needs. So, read on to learn more about the different methods of Intermittent Fasting.

16/8 Method

If you follow this method of Intermittent Fasting, you must fast for 16 hours daily. If you fast for 16 hours, the eating window comes down to 8 hours. You can squeeze in two or three healthy meals within this time frame. It is popularly known as the LeanGains method. The creator of this variant of Intermittent Fasting was Martin Berkhan, a fitness expert. This method can be something as simple as skipping your breakfast and directly having your first meal at noon and your last one at about 8 p.m.

The next meal you can have will be on the following day at noon. So, you will fast for 16 hours and, frankly, you will not even feel like you were fasting for 16 hours. Ideally, women must not fast for more than 14 hours. If you like to wake up early and eat breakfast, then have a hearty breakfast, then you need to make sure that your last meal is at around 4 or 6 in the evening.

You are free to consume all sorts of calorie-free beverages throughout the day like water, black coffee or any other herbal teas. You need to make sure that you don't include any sugar in your drinks, since it will effectively break your fast. If you want to lose weight, then you must not binge on junk foods when you break your fast. This method works, only if you strictly follow the protocols of the diet.

The 5:2 Diet

In this variation of the diet, you need to restrict your calorie intake on two days of the week and eat like you normally do on the other days. On the days you need to restrict your calorie intake, the calories you consume must be between 500 and 600. Michael Mosley is the creator of this diet and it is also known as the Fast diet. On the days that you fast, you must ensure you don't consume more than 600 calories. You can squeeze in two small meals within this calorie limit. This diet is ideal for all those who don't like the idea of fasting daily.

Eat-stop-Eat

In this form of Intermittent Fasting, you must fast for 24 hours, once or twice in a week. Brad Pilon, a famous fitness expert, created this diet.

You can choose the days you want to fast on. For instance, if your fast starts at 8 p.m. on Monday night, then you will break your fast only at 8 p.m. on Tuesday night. You can decide when you want to fast, if you fast for 24-hours. You cannot consume any solid food during your fasting period but can have calorie-free beverages. You must ensure that you are consuming healthy meals on the normal days. If you are just getting started with fasting, then this might be a little complicated. Instead, it is a good idea to start with either of the previous methods and then make your way toward this dieting protocol. If you want to follow this diet, then you need self-discipline and self-control.

Make sure that your fasting period never exceeds 48 hours. So, don't try to fast on two days continuously and pace it evenly.

Alternate Day Fasting

If you want to follow this method of Intermittent Fasting, then you need to consume 500 calories on every alternate day. If you are not a fan of a strict diet, then this will work well for you. You can eat like you normally do on all days except for the ones with the calorie restriction.

Warrior Diet

Ori Hofmekler, a famous fitness expert, was the creator of this diet. In this method, you need to have small portions of raw fruits and vegetables during the day and end your day with a hearty meal at night. You will essentially be fasting throughout the day and will feast at night. The eating window in this method is restricted to about 4 hours. The food that you can consume on this diet is quite like the food you can consume while following a Paleo diet. So, you are free to fill up on foods that are unprocessed. It essentially means that you can eat only those foods that our cavemen ancestors had access to. If you feel like your caveman ancestors could not have eaten something, then neither can you. If you don't want to fast all day long, you can snack on fruit and vegetables. It will keep your hunger pangs at bay.

Spontaneous Fasting

As the name suggests, you merely need to skip meals spontaneously. There is no fixed plan. If you don't feel like eating, you simply need to skip a meal. There will be times when you don't have time to eat or when you don't feel like eating. So, whenever you skip a meal, you are effectively following the protocols of this diet. It will not do your body any harm if you skip meals from time to time.

Chapter Three:
Benefits of Intermittent Fasting

Perhaps the most common reason why people opt for Intermittent Fasting is to lose weight. Apart from weight loss, there are various other benefits this diet offers, and you will learn about them in this chapter.

Weight loss

Intermittent Fasting alternates between periods of eating and fasting. If you fast, naturally your calorie intake will reduce, and it also helps you maintain your weight loss. It also prevents you from indulging in mindless eating. Whenever you eat something, your body converts the food into glucose and fat. It uses the glucose immediately and stores the fat for later use. When you skip a few meals, your body starts to reach into its internal stores of fat to provide energy. As soon as your body starts burning fats due to the shortage of glucose, you will start to lose weight. Also, most of the fat that you lose is from the abdominal region. If you want a flat tummy, then this is the perfect diet for you.

Sleep

Lack of sleep is a primary cause of obesity. When your body doesn't get enough sleep, the internal mechanism of burning fat suffers. Intermittent Fasting regulates your sleep cycle and, in turn, it makes your body effectively burn fats. A good sleep cycle has different physiological benefits - it makes you feel energetic and elevates your overall mood.

Resistance to illnesses

Intermittent Fasting helps in the growth and the regeneration of cells. Did you know that the human body has an internal mechanism that helps repair damaged cells? Intermittent Fasting helps kickstart this mechanism. It improves the overall functioning of all the cells in the body. So, it is directly responsible for improving your body's natural defense mechanism by increasing its resistance to diseases and illnesses.

A healthy heart

Intermittent Fasting assists in weight loss, and weight loss improves your cardiovascular health. A buildup of plaque in blood vessels is known as atherosclerosis. This is the primary cause for various cardiovascular diseases. Endothelium is the thin lining of blood vessels and any dysfunction in it results in atherosclerosis. Obesity is the primary problem that plagues humanity and is also the main reason for the increase of plaque deposits in the blood vessels. Stress and inflammation also increase the severity of this problem. Intermittent Fasting tackles the buildup of fat and helps tackle obesity. So, all you need to do is follow the simple protocols of Intermittent Fasting to improve your overall health.

A healthy gut

There are several millions of microorganisms present in your digestive system. These microorganisms help improve the overall functioning of your digestive system and are known as gut microbiome. Intermittent

Fasting improves the health of these microbiome and improves your digestive health. A healthy digestive system helps in better absorption of food and improves the functioning of your stomach.

Tackles diabetes

Diabetes is a serious problem on its own. It is also a primary indicator of the increase in risk factors of various cardiovascular diseases like heart attacks and strokes. When the glucose level increases alarmingly in the bloodstream and there isn't enough insulin to process this glucose, it causes diabetes. When the body is resistant to insulin, it becomes difficult to regulate the insulin levels in the body. Intermittent Fasting reduces insulin sensitivity and helps tackle diabetes.

Reduces inflammation

Whenever your body feels there is an internal problem, its natural defense is inflammation. It doesn't mean that all forms of inflammation are desirable. Inflammation can cause several serious health conditions like arthritis, atherosclerosis and other neurodegenerative disorders.

Any inflammation of this nature is known as chronic inflammation and is quite painful. Chronic inflammation can restrict your body's movements too. If you want to keep inflammation in check, then Intermittent Fasting will certainly come in handy.

Promotes cell repair

When you fast, the cells in your body start the process of waste removal. Waste removal means the breaking down of all dysfunctional cells and proteins and is known as autophagy. Autophagy offers protection against several degenerative diseases like Alzheimer's and cancer. You don't like accumulating garbage in your home, do you?

Similarly, your body must not hold onto any unnecessary toxins. Autophagy is the body's way of getting rid of all things unnecessary.

Chapter Four:
What to Avoid During a Fast

Intermittent Fasting helps rectify and reverse several health conditions, but it doesn't mean that it is ideal for everyone. An important thing that you need to keep in mind is that you need to consult your medical practitioner before you start this diet.

Who can fast?

The following people can fast

Healthy adults

All healthy adults can fast. It helps cleanse the body and there aren't any reasons why a healthy adult cannot fast.

Children

Usually, it isn't suitable for children up to the age of 18 to fast; however, children can fast. A child must only fast for a short duration and must not fast for prolonged periods. A perfectly healthy child doesn't have to fast. The general exception to this rule is all those who suffer from obesity. A child needs plenty of nutrition for growth and their body needs nourishment constantly. If the child is less than 18 years, please consult a medical practitioner.

Type-2 diabetes

Fasting helps reverse the harmful effects of type-2 diabetes. If you suffer from this, then you are free to fast. Before you start any diet, you must always consult your medical practitioner.

Who Cannot Fast?

Pregnant women

As such, there is no conclusive proof that shows the effect of Intermittent Fasting on a fetus. It is better to abstain from any diets if you are pregnant or are trying to conceive. If you are planning to start a family, then your body needs plenty of nutrition and you must not restrict your diet at this point of time. Also, mothers who are breast-feeding need to abstain from Intermittent Fasting. Fasting reduces the nutrition available in breast milk and it also affects the quantity of milk that is produced.

Any medical conditions

If you have any health concerns related to the kidney or the liver, then you must not fast. You need to consult a doctor before you fast if you have any pre-existing medical conditions. If you use any medication for high blood pressure or have a weak immune system, then you must not fast. You can fast even if you have medical conditions, but don't forget to consult your doctor.

If you have recently had a major surgery, then please abstain from fasting. Also, fasting is not ideal for all those who are recovering from any major illness.

Eating disorders

If you have any eating disorders or are recovering from an eating disorder, then you must not fast. Fasting can cause a relapse and you need to avoid it at any cost.

Afraid to fast

If fasting scares you, then don't fast. Fear is an unnecessary stressor and it will just cause problems. Fear is a powerful emotion and can alter your psychological makeup. If you think you cannot handle fasting, then don't try to fast. If you want this diet to generate positive results, you need to have an open mindset!

Foods to Avoid and Eat

When you are following the protocols of Intermittent Fasting, the primary focus is not on what you eat, but it is on when you eat. Just because it doesn't focus on what you eat, it doesn't mean that you stuff yourself with carbs and sugar-laden treats. For best results, it is a good idea to stay away from all processed foods and opt for healthy foods. It means that it is a good idea to avoid all sugary treats or at least try to limit them as much as you possibly can. So, avoid cookies, chocolates, cakes, and all packaged sweets.

Stay away from foods rich in unhealthy fats and carbs like burgers, pizzas and all fast foods. Say no to foods that are devoid of all protein and are full of sugars and carbs. Avoid soy products if you want to lose weight. Soy products are rich in estrogen and a high level of estrogen will not do you any good.

You need to maintain a calorie deficit if you want to lose weight. The higher the level of insulin in your body, the less fat you will lose. Carbs and sugars increase the level of insulin. So, if you want to regulate your insulin levels, you need to avoid carbs.

There are some people who believe that you can eat a lot of protein, fruit and vegetables while fasting. If you eat all this during a fast, you aren't effectively fasting, are you? Even if you had a couple of drops of honey to your morning tea, you will be effectively breaking your fast. Just because you aren't permitted to eat anything, doesn't mean that you stop drinking water.

Your body needs at least 8 glasses of water to stay hydrated and ensure that you are thoroughly hydrated. Drinking water will make you feel fuller and helps you to avoid any hunger pangs.

You are free to consume all calorie-free beverages like black tea, black coffee, green tea, herbal teas and carbonated water. Try to limit your caffeine intake. Caffeine has a diuretic effect on the body and too much of it can cause dehydration due to the loss of electrolytes. Try to limit your caffeine intake to about two cups of coffee or any other caffeinated calorie-free drink of your choice. It might seem quite tempting to add some sugar or cream to your coffee, or perhaps some honey to your tea. If you do this, you will cause a spike in your insulin levels. When there is a spike in your insulin levels, your body stops burning fat and it negates the benefits of fasting. You must try to avoid anything that will cause a spike in your insulin levels and effectively break your fast. Some people believe that chewing sugar-free gum will keep hunger at bay. Even all those products that are labeled as "no sugar" or "sugar-free" include some carbs in them.

If you really want to lose weight and want to improve your overall health, then it is a good idea to stay away from all forms of alcoholic drinks as well.

Alcohol contains a lot of carbs that can sneak up on you unknowingly. Intermittent Fasting helps cleanse your body. So, if you really want to cleanse your body then you need to avoid all the things that will result in the internal buildup of toxins. So, stay away from alcohol to improve the efficiency of this diet.

Intermittent Fasting

Table of Contents

Introduction

D o you want a diet that will help you lose weight and improve your overall health? Do you want a diet that doesn't prescribe calorie counting? It does sound quite wonderful if you can achieve your weight loss and health goals without counting calories, doesn't it? If your answer is yes, then you are in for a pleasant surprise! Intermittent Fasting is the diet that you have been looking for. Fasting is not a new concept and has been around for a long time. Intermittent Fasting is a simple variation of fasting and is very helpful. This dieting protocol alternates between periods of fasting and eating.

In this book, you will learn about the basics of Intermittent Fasting, the changes that take place in your body, the benefits it offers, different methods of Intermittent Fasting, tips to exercise, common FAQs and much more. Intermittent Fasting is quite simple. You merely need to make a couple of changes to your eating habits and you are good to go.

If you are fascinated by this diet and want to learn more about it, then let us start right now!

Chapter One:

History of Intermittent Fastin

U nlike other forms of conventional dieting, the concept of fasting is quite unambiguous and easy to understand. Did you know that most of us tend to unconsciously follow the protocols of Intermittent Fasting? Do you ever skip having breakfast or dinner? If you do, then you are following an Intermittent Fasting protocol. You will learn about the different methods of Intermittent Fasting in the coming chapters.

Our hunter and gatherer caveman ancestors had to seek food in nature. So, they were often on a fast until they found some nourishment. Then agriculture was introduced, and it led to the formation of human civilization. Whenever there was food scarcity or whenever the seasons changed, fasting was the norm. They used to maintain stocks of grain and meat in cities and castles for harsh winters. Before the introduction of agriculture, shortage of rainfall meant a spell of famine and people used to fast to make their food supplies last longer. Enough rain was quintessential to meet the grain requirement.

Along with civilizations, there came religions. Religions grew when people were living in close quarters and shared similar beliefs. Most of the religions prescribe fasting. Hinduism refers to fasting as Vaasa, and Hindus observe it during festivals or other auspicious days. Fasting is also considered to be a form of penance. Islam prescribes fasting during the holy month of Ramzan. A similar practice is present in Judaism and is known as Yom Kippur. There's a period of fasting before Easter in the Catholic faith.

Technology and innovations play a vital role in the evolution of humans. Industrialization revolutionized the food industry. Mass production of food products meant that the markets were constantly flooded with food products. Apart from this, the way humans view and consume food has also undergone a major change. The human body didn't get a chance to sufficiently adapt itself to the rampant changes brought about by industrialization and agriculture. All this meant that a host of health problems soon followed. Intermittent Fasting is quite an old practice. Even though it is an old practice, humans have just begun to understand and truly appreciate the various benefits this diet offers. Whenever you fast, you give your body a chance to cleanse itself - not just cleanse but even repair and regenerate itself from within.

Essentially, while fasting your body gets to burn out all the excess fat it has stored. Human beings have evolved in such a manner that we can fast without any health risks and that is normal. Body fat is the reserve of food that the body has stashed away for a rainy day. If you don't consume food, your body will simply reach into this reserve to provide you with energy. There needs to be balance in everything you do. There's a yin and a yang. The same rule applies to eating and fasting as well. Fasting is the flip side of eating. If you aren't eating, then you are fasting. When you eat something, this leads to an accumulation of food energy that isn't going to be made use of immediately. A portion of this is stored away. A hormone known as insulin is responsible for storing the food energy. When you eat something, there is a spike in the level of insulin. This facilitates the storage of energy in two different ways. Sugars are linked into long chains and this is known as glycogen. The rest is stored in the liver. When the space available has been maxed out, the liver starts turning the rest into fat. Some of this fat so created is stored in the liver and the rest is stored in the form of fat cells in the rest of your body. There isn't a limit on fat creation. So, there are two forms of energy stores in our bodies. One is easily accessible and has a limited storage space (glycogen), and the other is the harder to reach energy without a limit on storage (body fat).

This process is essentially reversed when you don't eat, that is during fasting. There will be a reduction in the level of insulin and this enables your body to reach into its storage of fat cells and burn this to provide energy. The most easily attainable source of energy for your body is glycogen. This is broken down into molecules of glucose that sustains your body. This can provide sufficient energy for your body to function for 24 hours or longer. After this, your body will reach into its fat reserves to generate energy. Your body will do this only while feeding or fasting. Either your body will be storing energy, or it will be burning energy. Only either of these processes can take place at any given time. If there is a balance between eating and fasting, then there will not be any weight gain. Over a period of time, you will start gaining weight if you haven't given your body sufficient time to burn all the food it has stored. To restore balance, you will need to give your body sufficient time to burn the food energy. This can be accomplished by fasting. This is how our bodies are designed. Intermittent Fasting helps to restore this much-needed balance.

Circadian Rhythm and Intermittent Fasting

Human beings, like other organisms, have a biological circadian clock that ensures that the physiological processes in the body are performed at the right time. The circadian rhythm is on all day long and it affects the biology and the behavior of humans. Any disruption in this rhythm has a negative effect on the metabolism and it can cause several metabolic dysfunctions like obesity, diabetes and a host of cardiovascular diseases. The primary factor that affects the circadian rhythm is the signal to eat. It is responsible for metabolic, physiological and behavioral pathways in the body. All these pathways are responsible for making sure that your body performs optimally. Apart from this, they also ensure that your body is healthy. You can use behavioral intervention to regulate the body's circadian rhythm. Yes, you guessed it right! Intermittent Fasting is a means of behavioral intervention that will streamline the circadian rhythm. This in turn leads to better gene expression and improvement in your body's health and metabolism.

Gut Microbiome and Intermittent Fasting

The gastrointestinal tract regulates multiple processes within your body. In other words, your gut helps regulate different physiological and biochemical functions in your body. For instance, the metabolic reaction to glucose and the blood flow are higher during the day than at night. Even a small fluctuation in the circadian rhythm can impair your metabolism and increases the risk of several chronic diseases. The microbiome present in the gut is usually referred to as the second brain. It is known as the second brain because of the influence it has over your metabolism and physiology. Intermittent Fasting has a positive impact on the gut microbiome. It makes the gut less permeable, reduces the chances of systemic inflammation and improves overall energy balance.

Lifestyle Behavior and Intermittent Fasting

Intermittent Fasting helps change different health-related behaviors like calorie consumption, energy expenditure and your sleep cycle. Therefore, it is not a surprise that these are the three primary functions that help fight the most significant health concern that plagues the human community, obesity. You will learn more about the different benefits it offers in the coming chapters.

Chapter Two:
Different Methods of Fasting

I ntermittent Fasting is a varied and a dynamic diet that offers multiple health benefits. There are different methods of Intermittent Fasting that you can follow, and you need to select one that will meet your needs. So, read on to learn more about the different methods of Intermittent Fasting.

16/8 Method

If you follow this method of Intermittent Fasting, you must fast for 16 hours daily. If you fast for 16 hours, the eating window comes down to 8 hours. You can squeeze in two or three healthy meals within this time frame. It is popularly known as the LeanGains method. The creator of this variant of Intermittent Fasting was Martin Berkhan, a fitness expert. This method can be something as simple as skipping your breakfast and directly having your first meal at noon and your last one at about 8 p.m.

The next meal you can have will be on the following day at noon. So, you will fast for 16 hours and, frankly, you will not even feel like you were fasting for 16 hours. Ideally, women must not fast for more than 14 hours. If you like to wake up early and eat breakfast, then have a hearty breakfast, then you need to make sure that your last meal is at around 4 or 6 in the evening.

You are free to consume all sorts of calorie-free beverages throughout the day like water, black coffee or any other herbal teas. You need to make sure that you don't include any sugar in your drinks, since it will effectively break your fast. If you want to lose weight, then you must not binge on junk foods when you break your fast. This method works, only if you strictly follow the protocols of the diet.

The 5:2 Diet

In this variation of the diet, you need to restrict your calorie intake on two days of the week and eat like you normally do on the other days. On the days you need to restrict your calorie intake, the calories you consume must be between 500 and 600. Michael Mosley is the creator of this diet and it is also known as the Fast diet. On the days that you fast, you must ensure you don't consume more than 600 calories. You can squeeze in two small meals within this calorie limit. This diet is ideal for all those who don't like the idea of fasting daily.

Eat-stop-Eat

In this form of Intermittent Fasting, you must fast for 24 hours, once or twice in a week. Brad Pilon, a famous fitness expert, created this diet.

You can choose the days you want to fast on. For instance, if your fast starts at 8 p.m. on Monday night, then you will break your fast only at 8 p.m. on Tuesday night. You can decide when you want to fast, if you fast for 24-hours. You cannot consume any solid food during your fasting period but can have calorie-free beverages. You must ensure that you are consuming healthy meals on the normal days. If you are just getting started with fasting, then this might be a little complicated. Instead, it is a good idea to start with either of the previous methods and then make your way toward this dieting protocol. If you want to follow this diet, then you need self-discipline and self-control.

Make sure that your fasting period never exceeds 48 hours. So, don't try to fast on two days continuously and pace it evenly.

Alternate Day Fasting

If you want to follow this method of Intermittent Fasting, then you need to consume 500 calories on every alternate day. If you are not a fan of a strict diet, then this will work well for you. You can eat like you normally do on all days except for the ones with the calorie restriction.

Warrior Diet

Ori Hofmekler, a famous fitness expert, was the creator of this diet. In this method, you need to have small portions of raw fruits and vegetables during the day and end your day with a hearty meal at night. You will essentially be fasting throughout the day and will feast at night. The eating window in this method is restricted to about 4 hours. The food that you can consume on this diet is quite like the food you can consume while following a Paleo diet. So, you are free to fill up on foods that are unprocessed. It essentially means that you can eat only those foods that our cavemen ancestors had access to. If you feel like your caveman ancestors could not have eaten something, then neither can you. If you don't want to fast all day long, you can snack on fruit and vegetables. It will keep your hunger pangs at bay.

Spontaneous Fasting

As the name suggests, you merely need to skip meals spontaneously. There is no fixed plan. If you don't feel like eating, you simply need to skip a meal. There will be times when you don't have time to eat or when you don't feel like eating. So, whenever you skip a meal, you are effectively following the protocols of this diet. It will not do your body any harm if you skip meals from time to time.

Chapter Three:

Benefits of Intermittent Fasting

Perhaps the most common reason why people opt for Intermittent Fasting is to lose weight. Apart from weight loss, there are various other benefits this diet offers, and you will learn about them in this chapter.

Weight loss

Intermittent Fasting alternates between periods of eating and fasting. If you fast, naturally your calorie intake will reduce, and it also helps you maintain your weight loss. It also prevents you from indulging in mindless eating. Whenever you eat something, your body converts the food into glucose and fat. It uses the glucose immediately and stores the fat for later use. When you skip a few meals, your body starts to reach into its internal stores of fat to provide energy. As soon as your body starts burning fats due to the shortage of glucose, you will start to lose weight. Also, most of the fat that you lose is from the abdominal region. If you want a flat tummy, then this is the perfect diet for you.

Sleep

Lack of sleep is a primary cause of obesity. When your body doesn't get enough sleep, the internal mechanism of burning fat suffers. Intermittent Fasting regulates your sleep cycle and, in turn, it makes your body effectively burn fats. A good sleep cycle has different physiological benefits - it makes you feel energetic and elevates your overall mood.

Resistance to illnesses

Intermittent Fasting helps in the growth and the regeneration of cells. Did you know that the human body has an internal mechanism that helps repair damaged cells? Intermittent Fasting helps kickstart this mechanism. It improves the overall functioning of all the cells in the body. So, it is directly responsible for improving your body's natural defense mechanism by increasing its resistance to diseases and illnesses.

A healthy heart

Intermittent Fasting assists in weight loss, and weight loss improves your cardiovascular health. A buildup of plaque in blood vessels is known as atherosclerosis. This is the primary cause for various cardiovascular diseases. Endothelium is the thin lining of blood vessels and any dysfunction in it results in atherosclerosis. Obesity is the primary problem that plagues humanity and is also the main reason for the increase of plaque deposits in the blood vessels. Stress and inflammation also increase the severity of this problem. Intermittent Fasting tackles the buildup of fat and helps tackle obesity. So, all you need to do is follow the simple protocols of Intermittent Fasting to improve your overall health.

A healthy gut

There are several millions of microorganisms present in your digestive system. These microorganisms help improve the overall functioning of your digestive system and are known as gut microbiome. Intermittent Fasting improves the health of these microbiome and improves your digestive health. A healthy digestive system helps in better absorption of food and improves the functioning of your stomach.

Tackles diabetes

Diabetes is a serious problem on its own. It is also a primary indicator of the increase in risk factors of various cardiovascular diseases like heart attacks and strokes. When the glucose level increases alarmingly in the bloodstream and there isn't enough insulin to process this glucose, it causes diabetes. When the body is resistant to insulin, it becomes difficult to regulate the insulin levels in the body. Intermittent Fasting reduces insulin sensitivity and helps tackle diabetes.

Reduces inflammation

Whenever your body feels there is an internal problem, its natural defense is inflammation. It doesn't mean that all forms of inflammation are desirable. Inflammation can cause several serious health conditions like arthritis, atherosclerosis and other neurodegenerative disorders.

Any inflammation of this nature is known as chronic inflammation and is quite painful. Chronic inflammation can restrict your body's movements too. If you want to keep inflammation in check, then Intermittent Fasting will certainly come in handy.

Promotes cell repair

When you fast, the cells in your body start the process of waste removal. Waste removal means the breaking down of all dysfunctional cells and proteins and is known as autophagy. Autophagy offers protection against several degenerative diseases like Alzheimer's and cancer. You don't like accumulating garbage in your home, do you? Similarly, your body must not hold onto any unnecessary toxins. Autophagy is the body's way of getting rid of all things unnecessary.

Chapter Four:

What to Avoid During a Fast

Intermittent Fasting helps rectify and reverse several health conditions, but it doesn't mean that it is ideal for everyone. An important thing that you need to keep in mind is that you need to consult your medical practitioner before you start this diet.

Who can fast?

The following people can fast

Healthy adults

All healthy adults can fast. It helps cleanse the body and there aren't any reasons why a healthy adult cannot fast.

Children

Usually, it isn't suitable for children up to the age of 18 to fast; however, children can fast. A child must only fast for a short duration and must not fast for prolonged periods. A perfectly healthy child doesn't have to fast. The general exception to this rule is all those who suffer from obesity. A child needs plenty of nutrition for growth and their body needs nourishment constantly. If the child is less than 18 years, please consult a medical practitioner.

Type-2 diabetes

Fasting helps reverse the harmful effects of type-2 diabetes. If you suffer from this, then you are free to fast. Before you start any diet, you must always consult your medical practitioner.

Who Cannot Fast?

Pregnant women

As such, there is no conclusive proof that shows the effect of Intermittent Fasting on a fetus. It is better to abstain from any diets if you are pregnant or are trying to conceive. If you are planning to start a family, then your body needs plenty of nutrition and you must not restrict your diet at this point of time. Also, mothers who are breast-feeding need to abstain from Intermittent Fasting. Fasting reduces the nutrition available in breast milk and it also affects the quantity of milk that is produced.

Any medical conditions

If you have any health concerns related to the kidney or the liver, then you must not fast. You need to consult a doctor before you fast if you have any pre-existing medical conditions. If you use any medication for high blood pressure or have a weak immune system, then you must not fast. You can fast even if you have medical conditions, but don't forget to consult your doctor.

If you have recently had a major surgery, then please abstain from fasting. Also, fasting is not ideal for all those who are recovering from any major illness.

Eating disorders

If you have any eating disorders or are recovering from an eating disorder, then you must not fast. Fasting can cause a relapse and you need to avoid it at any cost.

Afraid to fast

If fasting scares you, then don't fast. Fear is an unnecessary stressor and it will just cause problems. Fear is a powerful emotion and can alter your psychological makeup. If you think you cannot handle fasting, then don't try to fast. If you want this diet to generate positive results, you need to have an open mindset!

Foods to Avoid and Eat

When you are following the protocols of Intermittent Fasting, the primary focus is not on what you eat, but it is on when you eat. Just because it doesn't focus on what you eat, it doesn't mean that you stuff yourself with carbs and sugar-laden treats. For best results, it is a good idea to stay away from all processed foods and opt for healthy foods. It means that it is a good idea to avoid all sugary treats or at least try to limit them as much as you possibly can. So, avoid cookies, chocolates, cakes, and all packaged sweets.

Stay away from foods rich in unhealthy fats and carbs like burgers, pizzas and all fast foods. Say no to foods that are devoid of all protein and are full of sugars and carbs. Avoid soy products if you want to lose weight. Soy products are rich in estrogen and a high level of estrogen will not do you any good.

You need to maintain a calorie deficit if you want to lose weight. The higher the level of insulin in your body, the less fat you will lose. Carbs and sugars increase the level of insulin. So, if you want to regulate your insulin levels, you need to avoid carbs.

There are some people who believe that you can eat a lot of protein, fruit and vegetables while fasting. If you eat all this during a fast, you aren't effectively fasting, are you? Even if you had a couple of drops of honey to your morning tea, you will be effectively breaking your fast. Just because you aren't permitted to eat anything, doesn't mean that you stop drinking water.

Your body needs at least 8 glasses of water to stay hydrated and ensure that you are thoroughly hydrated. Drinking water will make you feel fuller and helps you to avoid any hunger pangs.

You are free to consume all calorie-free beverages like black tea, black coffee, green tea, herbal teas and carbonated water. Try to limit your caffeine intake. Caffeine has a diuretic effect on the body and too much of it can cause dehydration due to the loss of electrolytes. Try to limit your caffeine intake to about two cups of coffee or any other caffeinated calorie-free drink of your choice. It might seem quite tempting to add some sugar or cream to your coffee, or perhaps some honey to your tea. If you do this, you will cause a spike in your insulin levels. When there is a spike in your insulin levels, your body stops burning fat and it negates the benefits of fasting. You must try to avoid anything that will cause a spike in your insulin levels and effectively break your fast. Some people believe that chewing sugar-free gum will keep hunger at bay. Even all those products that are labeled as "no sugar" or "sugar-free" include some carbs in them.

If you really want to lose weight and want to improve your overall health, then it is a good idea to stay away from all forms of alcoholic drinks as well.

Alcohol contains a lot of carbs that can sneak up on you unknowingly. Intermittent Fasting helps cleanse your body. So, if you really want to cleanse your body then you need to avoid all the things that will result in the internal buildup of toxins. So, stay away from alcohol to improve the efficiency of this diet.

Chapter Five:

The Truth about Breakfast

L osing weight can be a little tricky at times. Do you want to know if you can speed up this process and effectively turn your body into a fat burning machine? If yes, then you need to start skipping breakfast. Yes, you read it right. You might think this isn't a good idea since breakfast is the most important meal of the day. Well, hold your horses before you jump to any conclusions. Go through the information given in this chapter and it will certainly change your beliefs about breakfast.

The human physiology is based on the feast-famine pattern of eating; the basic hunter-gatherer nature of our homo-sapien ancestors is still present within us. We might live in a modern world where there is dearth of food, but our bodies didn't have the necessary time to get used to this change. The constant dilemma that exists between modern society and our basic physiology is not a new problem. It isn't a good idea to ignore our basic physiology. Instead, you need to try to understand it so that you can do all that is necessary to make the most of your metabolism. If you want your body to work for you, then you need to take the time to understand how it works. You need to work with your metabolism and not against it, if you want to achieve your weight loss and health goals.

It is a popular belief that breakfast is the most important meal of the day. Almost all the popular weight-loss protocols recommend consuming a hearty breakfast. Another popular myth that we all seem to believe to be true is that skipping breakfast will cause obesity. Well, where did all these so-called truths come from? If you take a moment and think about it, these statements will not make any sense to you.

How can you even put on weight if you restrict your calorie intake? What is essential for weight loss? The answer is calorie deficit. So, if you skip breakfast, your body is in a calorie deficit and that must promote weight loss. So, doesn't it seem absurd to believe that skipping breakfast will make you gain weight?

So, it is nothing more than a myth and skipping breakfast will not make you fat. In fact, as per research published in 2014 in the *American Journal of Clinical Nutrition, this* showed that eating or skipping breakfast has no effect on weight loss.

When it comes to consuming food, the one thing you must never forget is to listen to your body. Your body is quite smart, and it knows what it wants. So, you must eat only when you are hungry. When your body needs food, it will let you know. If you don't feel hungry in the morning, then don't force yourself to eat breakfast and simply skip that meal. It is perfectly normal to skip breakfast and a lot of people do this.

Did you ever wonder why you don't feel hungry in the morning? The circadian system keeps our bodies in sync with the 24-hour format of day and night and our response to light and darkness. The Circadian system also affects your hormones, digestion and body temperature. Apart from this, it controls your hunger or appetite and is responsible for the lack of hunger in the morning and the hunger pangs in the evening. If you fast all night long, then you will not be hungry in the morning.

If there is a constant supply of glucose, then your body will not burn fat. Glucose is the easiest form of energy for your body and it will not tap into your fat reserves if you constantly give it glucose as a choice. If you keep consuming five or six meals a day, you will not burn any fats. You need to restrict your food intake if you want your body to burn fats.

All the food that you consume is converted into glucose and excess glucose is stored within the cells in the form of fat molecules. When you restrict your food intake for prolonged periods like you do while on Intermittent Fasting, then your body starts to reach into its fat stores to provide energy. You can optimize this process of burning fats by postponing your first meal of the day.

It is a common misconception that your body needs constant supply of glucose to function optimally. It might be true if you suffer from low sugar levels, but if you are healthy adult, then you don't have to worry about this. You don't have to keep eating after every couple of hours. If you keep feeding your body all the time, it starts to become resistant to insulin and it causes a whole range of health problems.

In fact, the most popular method of Intermittent Fasting- LeanGains, recommends that you skip breakfast. When you are asleep, your body keeps producing certain hormones that process fat and store some energy. So, as soon as you wake up in the morning, you will feel a burst of energy! This energy can keep you going for a couple of hours at least! You don't have to worry about skipping breakfast and it will certainly not harm you.

Chapter Six:

Frequency of Fasting

Intermittent Fasting is a pattern of eating that oscillates between periods of eating and fasting. There are a lot of myths about this method of fasting. In this chapter, let us debunk the most popular misconceptions that exist about fasting, snacking, and the frequency of eating.

Skipping breakfast will make you gain weight

Well, breakfast isn't as important as people seem to think. It might be thought of as the most important meal of the day, but it really isn't, and that notion is just a myth. People believe that skipping breakfast leads to excessive hunger and weight gain. There are no scientific studies or research that supports this claim. Skipping breakfast won't make you fat and you can do so quite safely without any fear. You can fast for 16 to 24 hours at a stretch without worrying about the functioning of your body. Your body knows what's best for it so trust your body.

Your metabolism improves when you eat frequently

It is a popular myth that eating frequently helps improve your metabolism. Eating small meals does not improve your body's ability to burn calories. Yes, your body does need some energy to digest and assimilate the food you consume. This is referred to as thermic effect of food and it accounts for about 20-30% of total calories from protein, 5-10% from carbs and about

3% from fats. On an average, the thermic effect of food accounts for 10% of the total calories you consume. You need to take into consideration the total calories you consume and not the number of meals you eat. You don't need to keep eating constantly. For instance, if you have three meals of 1000 calories each the thermic effect will be 300 calories and it will be the same if you have 6 meals of 500 calories each. So, you can fast for prolonged periods of time and not worry about slowing down your body's metabolism.

Eating frequently helps keep hunger at bay

People believe that snacking constantly helps to keep hunger at bay and reduces the chances of excessive hunger. Frequent meals will obviously leave you feeling full, but you don't have to do this. If you want to reduce your cravings and keep hunger at bay, then you need to make sure that you are filling yourself up with the right kind of food. Your meals must contain high amounts of fiber, protein and healthy fats instead of carbs. A meal that's rich in carbs will make you feel hungry soon and make you want to eat more food. Consuming carbs makes you crave for carbs. So, a balanced meal is the key to reducing your hunger. You don't have to worry about hungry pangs while following the protocols of Intermittent Fasting.

Small meals assist in weight loss

As mentioned earlier, frequent meals don't help boost your metabolism. Small meals won't do your body any good and they certainly don't help in weight loss. Eating frequently has the opposite of the desired effect. You can fast for an entire day without worrying about your body metabolism. There won't be a change in your energy levels if you keep snacking constantly. If you are worried that fasting leads to weight gain, you can lay those fears to rest. In fact, your body will start burning its reserves of fat to provide energy if you restrict the supply of glucose.

The brain needs glucose constantly

Yes, the brain does need glucose to function. This doesn't mean that you need to keep consuming carbs every couple of hours for our brain to keep functioning. It certainly won't stop functioning if you don't eat anything for an extended period. This misconception is due to the assumption that the brain needs glucose to function. Even if you restrict the consumption of food, your body can burn fats and produce energy that will keep your body going. Your body starts producing glucose that's necessary by a process known as gluconeogenesis. There is a reserve of glucose in the body and your liver breaks this down to supply glucose that is essential for the functioning of your brain. Even during the 24-hour format of fasting, your brain will function, and you don't have to worry about that. The dietary fats present in the body will be broken down into ketones by the liver for supplying the necessary energy your body needs. Ketones help in the functioning of the brain. Think about this from an evolutionary point of view. Human beings might have become extinct a long time ago if carbs were the only way for our survival. However, if an individual has hypoglycemia, then they will need to snack after every couple of hours if they don't want to get sick.

Eating often is necessary for good health

Being in a constantly fed state isn't natural for the human body. During evolution, humans had to endure periods of starvation. If eating often was essential for survival, then human beings might have been wiped out a long time ago. In fact, fasting helps to induce cellular repair by kick starting the process of autophagy. This helps to provide protection against diseases like

27

Alzheimer's and even certain types of cancer. Fasting is quite beneficial for the system and it helps cleanse the system by eliminating the build-up of toxins in the body. Snacking often has certain disadvantages as well. Frequent meals increase your calorie intake and lead to a build-up of fatty cells in the liver. This doesn't do your body any good.

"Starvation mode"

A popular argument against Intermittent Fasting is that it puts your body into starvation mode. While fasting, the body assumes that it's starving, and therefore shuts down its metabolism and prevents the burning of fat to produce energy. Long-term weight loss reduces the calories you burn and that's what starvation mode is. However, this is bound to happen regardless of the dieting protocol you follow. Short-term fasting helps speed up the metabolic function of the body. The increase in the levels of noradrenaline in the body increases the break down of the fat cells and thereby boosts the metabolism as well. Fasting for up to 48 hours helps boost the metabolism, but anything more than this reverses this effect. You can fast if you follow a sensible fasting protocol.

You will lose muscle while fasting

Once again, it is nothing more than a misconception that fasting leads to muscle loss. Fasting leads to fat loss and nothing else. In fact, Intermittent Fasting helps to increase the build-up of lean muscle and when coupled with the right exercises, it helps build muscle. Continuous calorie restriction for days on end leads to the loss of muscle. However, this isn't the case with Intermittent Fasting and you don't have to worry about losing muscle. You will learn more about building muscle in the coming chapters.

It is bad for your health

Some believe that fasting is harmful. Intermittent Fasting has several health benefits and these claims can be backed by scientific research. So, thinking that fasting is bad for overall wellbeing is nothing but a myth and it must not be taken seriously. In the previous chapter, the different health benefits of Intermittent Fasting were explained in detail. So, do you still think this diet is bad for you after going through the list of benefits it offers? Clearly this is just a myth and you must not pay any heed to it.

Intermittent Fasting leads to overeating

Some claim that Intermittent Fasting doesn't lead to weight loss and that instead it leads to overeating. After a fast, your consumption of food might be slightly higher. But this wears off quite quickly. Once your body gets acclimatized to prolonged periods of fasting, your calorie intake will start decreasing. You won't try to compensate for your fasting period by eating more during your eating window. Your body will slowly get used to fasting and you certainly don't have to worry about putting on weight.

Fasting certainly isn't bad for you and it can help improve your overall health. Depending on the Intermittent Fasting protocol that you opt for, your fasting schedule will change. You don't have to worry about the frequency of fasting, since your body will get the nutrients it needs to function properly.

Chapter Seven:

Gain Lean Muscle Mass

There has been an ongoing debate about whether it is good to exercise on an empty stomach or not. This heated debate has been going on since weights were introduced in gyms. As mentioned, it is a heated discussion and different people have different opinions. In this section, you will learn about how you can improve the efficiency of your workouts while on this diet.

One of the first things that we need to do is get some clarity about small and frequent meals. The popular opinion about eating smaller and frequent meals seems to be that it helps to speed up the metabolism and assists in burning fat. People also seem to think that it promotes the growth of muscle. You need to understand that there isn't the necessary research that supports these claims. Another idea that needs some clarification is whether it is a good idea to work out on empty stomach or not. The last question that needs some clarification is whether skipping meals will slow down your metabolism and increase the desire to eat.

You might wonder how you can clarify all these opposing opinions. Well, there are certain beliefs about Intermittent Fasting. You will learn about all these opinions and the facts related to these opinions that will help you. In this chapter, you will learn about exercising while following the protocols of Intermittent Fasting.

An empty stomach results in certain hormonal changes within your body that can promote the burning of stored fats and the building of muscle. An empty stomach increases your body's sensitivity to insulin and increases the production of growth hormones.

The Pancreas produces insulin in your body and it helps your body process the food that you consume. Insulin removes the blood sugar from your bloodstream and it transports it to the fat cells, muscles and liver for use later. The problem starts when you eat too much and too frequently, all this decreases the sensitivity of your body to insulin. A lower level of insulin sensitivity brings a host of health troubles like the inability to lose weight, gain weight, increase the fat content and increases the risk of several cardiovascular diseases along the way. If you eat less frequently, like you will while on Intermittent Fasting, it reduces the production of insulin and, therefore, lowers the risk of insulin sensitivity. The less insulin your body produces, the more sensitive it becomes to insulin and it helps burn the stored fat and reduces the risk of diabetes and cardiovascular disease.

When you exercise on empty stomach, your body pumps up the production of the magic elixir known as growth hormone that's necessary for the growth of muscles, stronger bones, longevity and for better fat burning. Some studies show that a 24-hour fast can increase the production of growth hormone in men by up to 2000% and by up to 1300% in women. These numbers seem quite unbelievable, don't they? All this by merely fasting for 24-hours.

You might be curious about the intermittent protocol and if it will affect your muscle mass. You will still be able to build muscle while following this diet. There are three things that you will need to keep in mind. Read on to learn more.

The Intermittent Fasting method that you might opt for will depend on the kind of a lifestyle that you are leading. Depending on your needs, whether spiritual or physical, you can select a specific method of fasting. Regardless of your reasons for starting on this diet, you might be wondering how you can build muscle while following the Intermittent Fasting protocols. It is a general misconception that you won't be able to build any muscle, but this cannot be further away from truth. There are a couple of things that you can do to maximize your success.

If you have a specific time when you are fasting, let's assume from 5 in the morning until 7 at night, then it is ideal if you can squeeze working out into your schedule during the evening hours. Waking up earlier than 5 a.m. isn't really possible. You will also need to eat before engaging in resistance training. So, working out in the middle of the day isn't advisable. You will need to consume proteins and carbs after working out to kickstart the recovery process. If you are training in the evening, then you can squeeze in a small meal after working out. You can work out for an hour and still give your body some time to recover before going to sleep.

You must plan your meals in such a way that the bulk of the calories you are supposed to consume is eaten right after your workout. It is important that you do this, because at this point your body will utilize all these calories to produce lean muscle mass and it will also facilitate in the recovery process. You will need to figure out the number of calories that you will need for building muscle. You will need to consume 20% of those calories prior to working out. The calories you consume must be a mix of proteins and carbohydrates. The other 60% of the total calories must be consumed in the period following your workout. You can spread this over two small meals if you want to and distribute it over the next couple of hours. Your calorie intake will definitely be high, and you can get in as many calories as you can by opting for foods that are rich in calories like oats, red meats and so on. Make sure that you are consuming foods that are rich in carbs after your workout. It will provide your body with the necessary calories to kick start the recovery process. You needn't worry about eliminating all fats from your meals. Instead, you can consume a large meal that's rich in carbs or proteins immediately after your training session and then have a high fat or protein meal just before you go to sleep. You must make it a point that your post-workout meal has low fat content. Fats are rich in calories and it is easier to have them in higher volumes (nuts, oils, and so on). It is certainly easier to have these than shoveling down carbs when you are already feeling full.

Finally, there is one more thing that you must keep in mind while following Intermittent Fasting protocols if you want to build some muscle. As soon as you wake up, you must eat something. If you are just fasting for the sake of convenience, then you must eat something according to your usual time of waking up in the morning. You must consume something just before your fast starts. Have some protein that can be digested slowly like red meat and cottage cheese. This meal must account for 20% of your daily calorie intake. A few carbs and fat can also be added to this meal. It will provide your body with the necessary amino acids to get through your fasting period. You have the option of going back to sleep if you feel like it. Having to wake up to eat and then going back to sleep is a hassle. This isn't something that will be sustainable in the long run. You must plan in such a manner that your body will get used to this schedule of eating. If you are used to waking up early in the morning, then this will be quite simple. You won't have to make any extra adjustments to your schedule. It will fit right in.

Make sure that you keep these tips in mind. If you try to engage in high intensity workouts while maintaining a low-calorie intake due to prolonged periods of fasting, this idea is likely to backfire. You will end up tiring yourself and your body will not have the necessary glucose to start the recovery process. After a while, your body will be depleted of glycogen and this will not do you any good. To prevent this, you will need to get used to eating forcefully. Your body will get used to this after a while, and it will start feeling normal. So, be patient and give yourself some time to get used to it.

Chapter Eight:
How to Get Started

Well, now that you know what Intermittent Fasting is all about and how it works, the next step is for you to get started with this diet. Intermittent Fasting is not merely a dieting protocol, but it is a way of life. Intermittent Fasting is sustainable in the long run and isn't a short-term diet. If you want to achieve and maintain your weight loss and overall health, then you must stick to this diet. Intermittent Fasting will help you shed all those extra kilos you want to lose. In this section, you will learn about the different steps that you can follow to get started on this diet.

Staring a new diet might seem slightly intimidating, but with the help of these steps, it will not seem intimidating.

Step One: Select a Method

There are various types of Intermittent Fasting protocols that you can choose from. One of the most versatile patterns of dieting these days is Intermittent Fasting. You need to opt for a method that fits your lifestyle, personality and meets your goals. If you are used to waking up early and like exercising, then the method of Intermittent Fasting that you can opt for is the 16:8 method. If you select this method, then you can have a breakfast in the morning and have your last meal in the evening. If you are used to skipping breakfast or don't mind skipping breakfast, then you can have your first meal at noon and your last meal at night. If you don't like the idea of fasting daily, then you can choose the alternate day fasting protocol and fast on alternate days. The method that you opt for is entirely up to you. You can customize this diet to meet your requirements. There is a method of fasting that will meet your requirements and you merely need to make up your mind about the method you want to opt for.

Step 2: Research

Go through all the information that is given in this book before you decide to select a specific method. Always select a method that suits your lifestyle. If you do this, it will be quite easy to stick to your dieting protocol. When compared to other conventional diets, this method is quite relaxed since Intermittent Fasting doesn't place much emphasis on what you eat but instead concentrates on when you eat. Check your priorities and find a method that will suit your needs. Once you establish your goals, you need to research about the fasting protocol you want to opt for. If you want to lose fat and gain lean muscle, then the method you must opt for is LeanGains.

Step 3: Find the necessary tools

There are various apps that you can use to help you with this diet. You can choose from free as well as paid applications to track your progress. Intermittent Fasting is essentially a method of trial and error. One method might be quite effective for some while something else might work for others. You can download an application that will help track your progress and determine whether a specific method is effective or not. If you want to, you can also maintain a food journal to track your progress. You need to make a note of when you eat and what you eat, along with the progress you are making.

Step 4: Starting the transition

Starting this diet might be a little tricky, if you don't have an all or nothing attitude. If you are used to skipping meals every now and then, then Intermittent Fasting will be quite simple. If you are not used to fasting and have never fasted before, then it will be a little difficult until you gain some footing. You need to prepare yourself mentally for the diet you want to follow. It might seem a little daunting that you need to go for prolonged periods without eating. Well, the one thing that you need to remember is that all your fears are baseless and, in fact, there is nothing that you need to fear. The fear is in your head and you will not get over it unless you take the first step.

You need to take some time to condition your body. To condition your body, you can slowly start increasing the gap between two meals. After you do this, you can start by slowly skipping a meal a day so that your body gets used to the idea of fasting. If you are used to snacking between meals, then you can slowly cut down on snacks. Instead, you can start filling yourself up with foods that will leave you feeling fuller for longer. After you do this, you can start with a relatively easy method of fasting. You can start with the alternate-day fasting method or the LeanGains method. It is all about slowly conditioning yourself to the diet and the idea of dieting. Once you do this, you will be able to follow the diet rather easily.

Step 5: Finding the necessary support

Everyone needs a support system. Your support system will encourage you and motivate you to keep going even when you feel like giving up. You can also start your diet with a diet buddy or partner. Find a partner for yourself and start the diet together. Your dieting buddy can be your partner, spouse, friend or anyone else. You can each use the other as a coach and a mentor along the way. If you cannot find someone to do this with, then you can explain your situation to someone and make them hold you accountable for the progress you make. Make that person check on you and the progress you are making.

Step 6: Toning down your workouts

You need to tone down your workout routine, at least initially. You need to give your body some time to get used to the new diet before you can go back to your exercise routine. When your body is getting used to a new diet, it is quite likely that you might feel a little low on energy. In such a situation, if you push yourself too hard, you risk burning yourself out and it will not do you any good.

Step 7: Following delayed gratification

Delayed gratification is a brilliant technique and it works rather well with this form of dieting. There might be times when a hunger pang strikes you and you might start craving for something sweet. Whenever this happens, make a list of the things that you want to eat. Keep adding the items to this list whenever you feel hungry. When this happens, you need to tell yourself that you cannot eat that right now and you can eat it later. When you do this, it helps to stop your mind about obsessing over things that you must not eat. You need to control your mind and you must not let it control you. You need to eat only those foods that are good for you.

Step 8: Protein must be a Priority

Always make sure that you eat the necessary proteins and complex carbs before anything else. You might have something sweet or oily on your eating list, but all that can wait. If you give in to your urge to eat something you aren't supposed to, then you will end up overeating. Also, it is quite likely that you will fill yourself up with junk during the eating window and then experience hunger pangs when you start fasting. When you are eating, you need to understand that you are prepping your body for the fasting period. So, you must always eat those foods that will leave you feeling fuller for longer like proteins, healthy carbs and dietary fats.

If you start feeling hungry while fasting, it is likely that you will give up on your diet. To avoid this, eat healthy and wholesome meals.

Avoid all sorts of processed foods that are full of sugars, unhealthy fats, and undesirable carbs. Instead, opt for healthy foods that are rich in fiber, nutrients, and the essential macros. Healthy food will nourish your body and will leave you feeling energetic. Unhealthy foods like chocolates or chips can be replaced with some fruits or nuts. Here are a couple of simple tips that you can keep in mind to make sure that you are eating wholesome food.

Have complex carbohydrates like whole grains and leafy vegetables instead of starchy foods like bread, pasta or pizza. Your meal must be rich in protein because it not only leaves you feeling fuller for longer, but it is good for you as well. Stay away from all processed foods and opt for healthy treats like kale chips, nuts, fruits, or anything that isn't full of saturated fats and trans fats. Replace sugary drinks with water (sparkling or still). Create a food plan for yourself. If you are interested in cooking, then learn to experiment with recipes and cook something different. Healthy food doesn't mean bland salads, so keep an open mind and try your hand at cooking. If you plan your meals in advance, then you can do all the meal prep on your day off, this does simplify the entire cooking process.

Step 9: Taking a "before" photograph

Before you start following any of the protocols of Intermittent Fasting, there is one little step along the way that you need to take. You need to take a photograph of yourself. You can label it as a "before" photograph. This will help you to get started. If you follow the protocols of Intermittent Fasting properly, then you will be able to see a positive change in your body. Keep taking a weekly photograph of yourself and make a timeline of the photographs. It will help you see the progress you are making. At times, you might need a little extra motivation to keep going. Whenever you hit a snag, you simply need to look at your timeline and it will provide you the necessary motivation to keep going. Also, keep a track of your body measurements. At times, you might not notice any weight loss, but you will be able to see a change in your body measurements.

Step 10: Things to keep in mind

If you are getting started with Intermittent Fasting or you want to try this diet, then there are a couple of things that you will need to keep in mind. You need to understand that the initial couple of days might be quite hard. Your body will take some time to get accustomed to the new diet and during this time, you need to fight your urge to give in. You need to stick to this diet for at least three weeks before you can see a visible change in your body. It can difficult to battle your hunger pangs until your body gets used to fasting. So, you need to come up with ways in which you can do so. You will learn more about the different tips that you can follow to make the diet easier in the next chapter.

Follow the simple steps given in this section to devise a plan of action to get started with this diet.

Chapter Nine:
Tips and Tricks

Well, now that you know what Intermittent Fasting is all about and the way you can get started, the next step will be to incorporate any of the Intermittent Fasting protocols into your life. In this chapter, let us look at a couple of tips that will come in handy while following the protocols of this diet.

Whenever you feel that a hunger pang is about to strike, take a couple of deep breaths and have a glass of water. The hunger pang must pass you by in less than 15 minutes. If it doesn't ease up, you can have a cup of green tea, herbal tea, or even black coffee.

Whenever you are breaking your fast, don't start gorging on food immediately. You must not try stuffing yourself with as much food as you possibly can but instead, take a couple of minutes and let the intense hunger pass before you start eating. There is no rush, so eat slowly and avoid all sorts of distractions. So, turn the TV off while eating and keep your phone switched off. Don't indulge in mindless eating and practice mindful eating. Enjoy what you are eating and indulge your senses. Don't try to compensate for the fasting period by stuffing yourself with food as you aren't doing yourself any good whatsoever.

It is ideal that you start your meal by having foods that are full of nutrients. So, fill up your plate with food rich in proteins, natural fats, and fiber, instead of carbs and sugars. Protein and fiber will help you feel fuller for longer and will reduce your calorie consumption as well. Nutrition must be your priority and not the quantity of food you consume. If you ever feel like having a cup of ice cream, make sure that you fill yourself up with nutritious food before indulging yourself with a sugary treat.

Try to keep yourself as busy as you possibly can be and don't sit idly. If you are always working, then you won't have any spare time to think about hunger or plan for your next meal. The more you think about food, the hungrier you will feel. Do your best to keep yourself busy.

Your body will take about a week or so to get used to any of the Intermittent Fasting protocols. Once your body is used to it, you can incorporate high-intensity workouts into your exercise schedule. Working out while you are fasting will help to improve the process of weight loss by speeding up the process of burning fats for fuel generation. However, observe caution while doing so. If you feel tired or even fatigued, you must immediately stop what you are doing. Make sure that you always keep your body hydrated.

You might overindulge during an initial couple of days of Intermittent Fasting. At least the first couple of times when this happens, don't panic and don't worry unnecessarily. It is just your body's survival instinct kicking in due to the absence of food. Your survival instinct is hardwired into your brain, and it will take a week or two to condition yourself. After a while, you will start eating regular-sized meals. So, don't worry.

During the eating window, you don't have to count calories and are indeed free to eat anything; however, this doesn't mean that you eat all sorts of junk. You must eat in such a manner that you will not be hungry during your fasting period. If you start feeling hungry immediately after a meal, you can always have a small snack. You must merely make sure that you are sticking to your fasting and feeding schedule.

You must always start out slowly. Remember that neither your body nor your mind is used to not eating for prolonged periods of time. It will take some time to condition yourself. You will be setting yourself up for failure if you think that you can immediately start fasting for 24 hours at a stretch. Instead, work on gradually increasing the gap between two meals. You can also begin by skipping one meal at a time.

You can maintain your blood sugar levels throughout the day by having high-quality carbohydrates like vegetables and fruit along with a lot of protein and naturally fatty food. It will also help your body optimize its ability to burn all the stored fat. Instead of having a meal that's full of carbs, make sure you are getting all the nutrients you need and not just the calories.

You must adjust your eating window in such a manner that your body gets a couple of hours to digest the food you eat before you can sleep at night. Don't go to bed the minute you have finished eating. At times, you might feel slightly hungry before you sleep. However, you must just let that hunger pang pass. You will feel quite full in a right way when you wake up in the morning.

Lack of sleep happens to be one of the significant obstructions to losing weight. So, make sure that you get good quality sleep at night. For optimal functioning of your body and brain, you need about 7 hours of undisturbed sleep daily.

At times, you might have to break your fast before the fasting period ends and it is okay. You don't have to beat yourself up for it. Occasionally, you can have a cheat day. However, make sure that neither of these things is a regular occurrence and just happens to be an isolated incident. Don't let it demotivate you and you must certainly not let it stress you out.

Your mind is the most significant hurdle

Implementing Intermittent Fasting is easy. When you eat depends on the form of Intermittent Fasting you decide to follow. If you want to fast daily, then it can be something as simple as giving your breakfast a miss when you wake up. Instead, you start your eating window with lunch and go about your day as usual. However, there is a mental barrier that you might come across. You might wonder how you can go through your day without breakfast. Do you feel that you will faint if you don't eat or that you will not be able to think straight? These questions are natural, and it is okay if you have any reservations about this diet. When you try this diet, you will understand that all these fears are unwarranted. Nothing will happen to your body if you don't eat one meal a day. In fact, you will feel better and more energetic than you ever did. If you keep thinking that you need to eat every couple of hours or have five meals daily or have your breakfast, or whatever it is that you have convinced yourself of, it is all in your mind. You believe all this because you were told it, not because you ever tried it for yourself. Your ability to think is essential. If you can think differently, you can act differently as well.

It is easy to lose weight

When you tend to eat less frequently, your overall food intake reduces. As a result of all this, you will end up losing weight while you follow Intermittent Fasting. You might plan for big meals but eating them consistently will not be easy. Intermittent Fasting is an excellent idea for all those who want to lose weight because it merely reduces your overall carb intake. Even if you have two large meals daily, the calories you eat will undoubtedly be less than when you ate six meals a day. By merely cutting down on how much you eat, you can lose weight. After all, it is quite simple

46

to lose weight. So, if weight loss is your primary aim, then you accomplish it with this simple diet.

If you want, you can build muscle

You can build muscle while you fast. You don't have to worry about losing muscle while on this diet. Also, the muscle you gain will be lean muscle. If you want a lean and toned body, then this is the best diet for you.

You can work while you fast

You will realize that you are more productive while you're on a fast. Your energy levels will be quite high when you wake up in the morning. The first three hours of the morning will be the most productive portion of the day for you. Well, that's about 12 to 15 hours into your diet, and that's when your body functions optimally. You might believe that your brain will not function optimally when it doesn't get necessary glucose. Well, all that's just a misconception. Since you no longer need to worry about what you can eat for breakfast, you can use this time to do something that's more productive. Your body produces energy while you sleep, and you can utilize this store of power as soon as you wake up. If you want to become productive, then you certainly must give this diet a go.

Cycle what you eat

Intermittent Fasting works well. However, you can make it more efficient by calorie and carb cycling. Do you know what these terms mean? You must have a couple of extra calories on the day you decide to exercise. So, you cycle calories by increasing your food intake. On the other days, you must aim for a calorie deficit. The idea behind this logic is quite simple. You can train to build muscle on all those days you exercise and, on the other days, you can encourage your body to burn fat. You must cycle your carbs on the day you train. It helps to stimulate the loss of fat. Have high protein and low-fat meals on regular days and the days you work out, have some carbs.

It is a lifestyle

We often tend to think of our diets as short-term regimes. It is better to be mindful of what you eat throughout the week instead of just a day or a couple of hours. Whether you have a protein shake 30 minutes before you work out isn't much of an issue if you have a high protein meal within 24-hours of your workout. Intermittent Fasting works because of the eating restriction it places on you. Let us say that you have three meals daily; it is a grand total of 21 meals in a week. Over the course of the diet, do you think your body cares if you eat from 8 a.m. to 8 p.m. in the day or from 1 p.m. to 1 a.m.? How about we stretch it out for a month? Would it make sense to have 80 well-balanced meals so that your body can make the most of it regardless of the time frame within which you eat? It is essential to understand that the food you eat usually has a great impact on your overall health. The diet will not make any sense if you starve yourself daily and then break your fast with all sorts of junk. It is better to think of Intermittent Fasting as a lifestyle choice instead of a mere diet. Not only does it make the diet more practical to follow, but you can maintain your weight loss as well. If you follow the diet religiously for two months and then go back to your unhealthy ways, it will not do your body any good. In fact, all the good that the diet did will be nullified.

You will want less food

When you fast, you will realize that your body craves less food. The diet doesn't victimize you. In fact, it teaches you to listen to your body. You will do what your body tells you to. While you fast, you might think of a hundred different things you want to eat, but when you break your fast, your opinion is bound to change. Once you get used to the diet, you will want to eat only when you are hungry. In a way, Intermittent Fasting curbs mindless eating.

Lose fat and gain muscle

If you want to lose fat and build lean muscle, then you must follow Intermittent Fasting, carb cycling and calorie cycling. It is not practically possible to lose gain muscle and even lose fat simultaneously. To lose weight, your body needs to burn more calories than you consume. So, it is essential to maintain a net calorie deficit to shed weight. However, if you want to build muscle, you need to consume more calories than you burn. It is apparent that you cannot have a net surplus and a net deficit simultaneously. For instance, you can either eat more than 2000 calories or less than 2000 calories at a given point in time. It is the reason why it is impossible to burn excess fat and gain muscle at the same time. However, if you don't think about the small timeframe and think about the diet over the course of a month instead of a day, you have more options available. For instance, you can decide to work out three days in a week, and you can maintain a calorie deficit on all the other days of the week. Therefore, your body will lose fat on a couple of days and gain muscle on the rest. But you cannot do both at the same time. So, you must think about your diet from a long-term perspective instead of a day-to-day diet.

More gains when you fast

There is a simple hypothesis for strength training, and it goes as follows "Always do the most important thing before the rest." It is about prioritizing. It works well not just for your diet, but with any other aspect of your life as well. It is quite simple. You must set one goal for your workout schedule, and you must do the exercises that are more important than others. For instance, let us assume that you work out three days in a week - Monday, Wednesday and Friday. You can do two sessions every session, the upper body workout and the lower body workout. The results you derive from exercise are more when you are fasting.

Fasted state

If you don't exceed 50 calories, your body will stay in a fasted state. There is no scientific evidence about whether it is true or not, but it seems to work for the majority. So, if you like to start your day with a glass of orange juice or a cup of coffee, then you can do so without any worry. Just make sure that your calorie intake doesn't exceed 50 calories. The idea of an intermittent fast is to switch your body to a fasted state instead of a fed state. It is quite easy, and you don't have to make any drastic changes to your daily schedule.

Drink lots of water

You must prepare yourself to drink plenty of water while you fast. Most of us aren't used to drinking a lot of water. In fact, we tend to forget that our body needs water. You can rectify this situation by drinking water. You must have at least eight glasses of water daily, and Intermittent Fasting will help you. Drinking plenty of water helps to detoxify your body and improves the health of your skin as well.

The best diet

Who would not want the ultimate diet plan? Everyone wants one. However, there is no such thing as a perfect diet. The diet that works well for one person might not work for someone else. Some might prefer the 24-hour method and others might like Leangains. The idea is to follow a diet that works well for you. If you want, you can try the different variations of Intermittent Fasting before you select one method. Your body isn't the same as someone else's, and its metabolism differs as well.

It is essential to stay motivated even when you don't seem to lose any weight while on an intermittent fast. So, you successfully made it through the first week or two of Intermittent Fasting, but you don't notice any weight loss? You will probably not see any fat loss within the first two weeks of the diet. Understand that this is normal and it doesn't mean that the diet isn't working for you. Fat loss starts only after three weeks of the diet. So, you need to keep going even when you feel like it's not working. Or maybe you are in a slump and cannot see the results that you once could. Well, it is important that you don't lose faith in the diet and that you keep going even when you don't want to. All that sounds simple, but how can you stay motivated? In this section, you will learn about a couple of simple steps that you can follow to make sure that you stay motivated and on the right track. If you give up now, all the efforts you put in until now will be for nothing.

While you follow Intermittent Fasting, you will feel quite energetic and sharp when you wake up in the morning. In fact, you will feel more energetic than ever. Your body will start to function optimally. The best part about this diet is that you can do everything like you normally would. Concentrate on how good you felt while on this diet, and it will motivate you. A little bit of self-control and self-discipline can help you stay on track. If you feel that a method isn't working for you, try another method and see is that works. Try different foods. It is a process of trial and error. So, don't give up just yet.

Chapter Ten:
Mistakes to Avoid

Now that you are aware of the protocols of Intermittent Fasting and the benefits it offers, you must be quite excited to get started! Before you start this diet, you need to be aware of a couple of common mistakes that you need to avoid. If you avoid the mistakes discussed in this chapter, then you can maximize the benefits you derive from this diet.

Mistake 1: Giving up too soon

Intermittent Fasting might not be easy during the initial weeks. You will need to go for prolonged periods of time without eating. Regardless of the method you opt for, you will need some discipline to ensure that you stick to your diet. During the initial week or two, you will need to combat your hunger pangs if you want this diet to be successful. If you can tough it out for a week or so, you will start to see the positive benefits of this diet. So, don't make the mistake of giving up too soon. Instead, trust the process and the diet and you will see positive results within no time.

Mistake 2: Binge Eating

When you break your fast, you might be tempted to stuff yourself with a lot of food. If you start overloading on calories after fasting for 16 hours, it will negate the benefits of this diet. If you indulge in binge eating whenever you break your fast, this diet will not do you any good. Instead, pace yourself and eat slowly. Your stomach takes about twenty minutes to realize when you are feeling full. So, take your time while eating and don't eat if you aren't hungry.

Mistake 3: Not eating enough

You need to eat until you are full and no more than that. If you don't eat anything at all, then you run the risk of starving yourself. If your body shifts into starvation mode, then you cannot achieve your weight loss and health goals. A lot of people worry that they will undo all that they have achieved while fasting if they eat during the eating window. If you do this, then it will be quite difficult to go through the subsequent spell of fasting. Your body needs food to function optimally. So, if you skip meals unnecessarily or if you don't eat enough food, you are merely hurting yourself.

Mistake 4: Wrong Foods

You need to eat the right foods if you want to lose weight or achieve your fitness goals on this diet. It isn't merely about the calories you consume, but about the quality of nutrition you feed your body. If you fast for 12 hours and then eat a tub of ice cream, it certainly will not do you any good! The way your body metabolizes food is quite different. For instance, if you consume 500-caloires of avocado it will be metabolized quite differently from 500 calories of cookies or chips! Also, if you end up eating junk food after breaking your fast, it is quite likely that you will be hungry within no time at all.

The protocols of Intermittent Fasting dictate that you need to eat a healthy and a well-balanced meal after breaking your fast! Ensure that you consume the necessary macros before you think about indulging in any junk food. Fill yourself up with protein and fiber-rich food, healthy dietary fats and some carbs before you even think about reaching for a chocolate bar.

Mistake 6: Forgetting to drink

You need to consume calorie-free beverages throughout the day to keep your body thoroughly hydrated. If you don't drink plenty of water and stay thirsty for long periods, it can trigger unnecessary hunger pangs. Usually, hunger pangs are a sign that your body is thirsty. Also, if you keep your body hydrated, you will feel satiated while fasting.

Mistake 7: Taking it too far

At times, you might not be able to fast for 16 hours at a stretch and you might want to break your fast earlier than usual. If that's the case, then please do so, but don't make a habit of it. You need to learn to listen to your body. Your body knows what it needs. Intermittent Fasting isn't about numbers. Instead, it is about doing what is good for your body. Don't take it too far and risk burning yourself out.

If you avoid the common mistakes discussed in this chapter, it will be quite easy to stick to Intermittent Fasting.

Chapter Eleven:

Intermittent Fasting and Weight Loss

Intermittent Fasting has become quite popular recently and it is an effective way of losing weight as well. This method of eating involves fasting for short periods of time. It helps to optimize the production of hormones that assist in controlling the weight. Fasting helps to reduce your calorie consumption. As mentioned in the previous chapters, there are different methods of Intermittent Fasting. The most popular ones happen to be the 16/8 method, eat-stop-eat method and the 5:2 diet. If you don't overeat during the non-fasting periods, you will be able to lose weight.

The effect of Intermittent Fasting on your hormones

The human body stores energy or calories in the form of body fat. Once you restrict your food intake or when you fast, there are several changes that take place in your body, for making this stored energy accessible. The changes in the activity of the nervous system also lead to changes in several important hormones in the body. When you start fasting, your insulin levels will decrease and it helps to burn fat. The production level of the human growth hormone (HGH) also increases. The norepinephrine that is released by the nervous system helps break down the fat stored in cells into fatty acids that help generate energy. Fasting for short periods of time will facilitate burning of fat. However, fasting for prolonged periods of time can suppress your metabolism. Therefore, Intermittent Fasting is a really good idea.

Helps in reducing calories and losing weight

Intermittent Fasting is effective since it helps reduce your calorie consumption. Regardless of the type of fasting method you opt for, you will need to fast for short periods of time. This will help to reduce your calorie consumption. A study that was published in 2014 showed that Intermittent Fasting over a period of 3-24 weeks could help reduce the body weight by 4-8%. The study also showed that people lost belly fat as well. The benefits offered by Intermittent Fasting aren't just restricted to weight loss. It has several metabolic benefits and it can help prevent a few chronic diseases as well. You needn't count calories on your normal eating days. However, on the fasting days make sure that you don't exceed 500-600 calories per day. Intermittent Fasting can easily help you restrict your calorie intake.

Holding on to muscle while you are dieting

When you start dieting, your body not only starts burning fat, but it starts burning muscle as well. There are several studies that show that Intermittent Fasting will help you burn fat without burning any muscle. In one study, it was discovered that the weight loss on Intermittent Fasting was the same as the weight loss that would have resulted from restricting calories for prolonged periods of time. However, there was hardly any reduction in the muscle mass.

Easier to eat healthy

The simplicity of this diet is one of its main advantages. Instead of eating three meals every day, you get to eat two or maybe three small meals every day. This makes things easier. Not only is this diet easy to follow, but it doesn't take much to stick to it either. You get to lose weight and maintain the weight loss over a long period of time.

There are different ways in which you can lose weight. Intermittent Fasting has become a popular method of fasting in the recent past. This method involves fasting for a short duration of time. Fasting for short periods of time will help people to consume fewer calories, and it also helps them optimize the hormones that regulate weight gain or loss. There are different methods of Intermittent Fasting to choose from, and you can opt for a technique that you feel is best suited for you. As long as you fast carefully and don't exceed your calorie intake or binge on junk food on non-fasting days, you are bound to drop those extra pounds.

Weight Loss

Your body stores away energy or calories in the form of body fat. When you don't consume anything, then your body will change several things within itself to make this stored energy available to it. It is all related to the changes in the activities performed by your central nervous system and also changes in the levels of various essential hormones in your body. When you fast, there are a few things that will change your metabolism such as the level of insulin changes when you fast. When you eat, insulin levels increase and when you fast it decreases. A low level of insulin will help burn away the accumulated fat. During a fast, Human Growth Hormone or HGH will increase, and this helps you to gain muscle and reduce fat. Fat cells are broken down into norepinephrine, and this helps in the burning down of fatty acids to generate energy. Despite the widespread belief that consuming five to six small meals is good, short-term fasting helps burn fat. Some studies suggest that fasting for 48 hours can help boost your metabolism and fasting for more than 48 hours can suppress the same. Short-term fasting can lead to several changes in your body and also the hormones that are produced.

Intermittent Fasting will also help you reduce calorie intake and help you lose weight. The reason for the success of Intermittent Fasting works is it reduces the number of calories that you are consuming. The different protocols that you will have to follow during the fasting periods make sure that you aren't eating more calories than those required by your body. If you follow Intermittent Fasting for three weeks, you will be able to see a change in your body and will have noticed a significant weight loss as well. With alternate day fasting, you can lose up to one 1.7 pounds every week. Intermittent fasting will also help you lose belly fat and will reduce your circumference. These results are indeed awe-inspiring and show that Intermittent Fasting is an excellent tool for assisting you to lose weight.

The benefits of Intermittent Fasting go well beyond just weight loss. It helps to improve your metabolism and will also help you prevent many chronic diseases while expanding your lifespan. Although you needn't count calories when you are on an Intermittent Fasting diet, overall weight loss usually depends on the reduction in the number of calories consumed. A particular study proves that Intermittent Fasting and continuous calorie restriction display the same results when compared amongst members belonging to similar groups. Intermittent Fasting is indeed a very convenient way of restricting the calories consumed without making any conscious effort of trying to eat less.

As mentioned in the previous chapters, Intermittent Fasting not only helps you lose weight but it will also help you hold on to muscle. One of the most prominent side effects of dieting on your body will be the burning of tissue along with fat. Intermittent Fasting can help you shed weight without any reduction in the muscle mass in your body. On a diet with just calorie restrictions, your body will start breaking down muscle to fuel itself. In calorie restriction diets about 25% of the weight loss was muscle mass, and in Intermittent Fasting diets only 10% of weight loss was associated with muscle mass. One study was conducted where the participants were all asked to consume the same amount of calories, except they had to do this in just one huge meal given to them in the evening. They not only lost body fat but also increased their muscle build up, along with a host of other beneficial changes in their health. However, there are a few limitations to the studies that were conducted, so you will probably take these findings with a pinch of salt. When compared to any standard diet you might have tried, Intermittent Fasting will help you hold onto your muscle mass while burning away all the unnecessary body fat.

If you want to succeed at Intermittent Fasting, then there are certain things that you must keep in mind if you're going to be able to lose weight. You will need to make sure that the food that you are consuming is of good quality and you must try eating whole foods whenever possible. You must not forget how important it is to count calories. Don't try to eat too "normally" on your non-fasting days, not so much that you end up compensating for the calories that you didn't consume on your fasting days. It is essential to be consistent. This rule applies to any weight loss method that you might try. You need to try it for a few weeks at least if you want it to work. It will take your body a while to get accustomed to this new fasting protocol. You need to be consistent with your meal schedule, and over a period, this will become easy.

Most of the Intermittent Fasting rules also recommend that you take up strength training. It is essential if you want to burn your body fat while you are still holding onto your muscle mass. During the initial week or two, you needn't bother counting the calories you consume, but after that, you need to be careful. If you feel like your weight loss has stalled, then you must reconsider your calorie intake. The requisites of Intermittent Fasting are that you eat a healthy diet and maintain a negative calorie count or deficit if you want to lose weight. You also must be consistent in your diet and don't forget to exercise.

Well, you need to remember that, at the end of the day, Intermittent Fasting is just a tool that you can make use of when you are trying to lose weight. The primary reason for this is the reduction in your calorie intake. There are specific definite effects essential hormones have on the body that contribute to the same. Intermittent Fasting might not be for everyone, but it might prove helpful if you try it out. So, try Intermittent Fasting for a few weeks, and you will be able to see the change for yourself.

The best way to lose weight is to lose primarily body fat, and when it comes to doing that, nothing beats the one-two knock out combination of proper diet, which we've already covered with the different Intermittent Fasting protocols, and exercise. Exercising helps you not just burn more calories but also helps maintain a fast metabolism – even develop a faster one, which is the ability to burn calories. In this section, we'll take a look at two ways to exercise for weight loss.

Resistance or Weight Training

One of the most popular misconceptions about this type of exercise, especially for women, is that it will lead to super big muscles that'll make ladies look like Dwayne "The Rock" Johnson or Terry Crews. Nothing can be further from the truth. Guys like them are freaks of nature. Even better, women bodybuilders are even rarer. Whether referring to men or women, only 1% of the population has the potential to grow muscles that are that big. Of course, it requires synthetic drugs like steroids too. Given that your chances of bulking up with muscle via resistance training alone are virtually zero, you can breathe normally now. The good news about weight training is instead of bulking up, it will help you reduce your size and you will become leaner. Resistance training, according to studies, can be more effective in burning body fat compared to cardio. It's because it helps maintain muscle mass – increase it even – and muscle mass is key to proper metabolism. Simply put, less muscle mass means a slower metabolism. But again, this doesn't say you'll have to be as big as the Incredible Hulk, Thor, Superman or Captain America.

Oh – and it helps firm and shape up your favorite body parts like the chest, butt and arms, among other parts.

Exercise and Intermittent Fasting will help you sculpt the body you always wished for.

Cardiovascular Training

If weight or resistance training is superior to cardiovascular training, why do you need to incorporate it into your weight loss efforts? For one, just because it's not as good doesn't mean it's worthless and doesn't help. The primary benefit of doing this type of training is that it helps make your heart and lungs stronger and more efficient regarding delivering much-needed blood and oxygen all through your body, which is key to better exercise performance and overall health. Another benefit is that it does help burn body fat, though not as much as resistance or weight training. And lastly, it's much easier to do given all you need is a good pair of running or brisk walking shoes and exercise clothes and you can hit the road for a run or walk, which isn't like weight or resistance training, which requires specialized equipment. While you can do bodyweight training, it's often too difficult for beginners.

You'll have to exercise caution when it comes to doing cardio work because if you do too much, your body will start to consume muscle tissue for energy instead of calories and body fat. And given that muscle mass is key to having proper metabolism, less muscle mass means slower metabolism – and less ability to burn body fat. So how much is too much? More than 45 straight minutes of regular cardio and more than 30 consecutive minutes of high-intensity cardio is too much.

Exercise Intensity and Duration

The thread that runs through both resistance and cardio training, particularly when it comes to optimal weight loss, is intensity. Simply put, it means the amount of effort put in.

There are three intensity levels when it comes to exercising – low, moderate and high. The optimal intensity is moderate.

So how do you find out your current exercise intensity level? The most straightforward and relatively accurate way of doing so is called the talk test. After exercising for a couple of minutes, try talking as you continue exercising. If you can still carry on a very normal conversation with no effort whatsoever, it means you're exercising at low intensity, which means it's too easy to burn any significant amount of calories. If you can barely talk or carry on a conversation normally, huffing and puffing throughout, your intensity is high, i.e., too hard. If you can still carry on with a normal conversation, but with some effort or strain in breathing or talking, that's moderate intensity – the perfect intensity for optimal fat burning. Moderate intensity must be maintained for a specific period. Otherwise, it won't help you burn significant calories for weight loss. Exercise for too long puts you at risk of losing muscle mass and for too short a period, at risk of being unable to burn many calories. The optimal window is between 20 to 45 minutes of moderate intensity exercise.

Follow the simple exercising tips given in this chapter to speed up the process of weight loss.

Chapter Twelve:

Intermittent Fasting While Travelling

U p until now, you were introduced to different methods of Intermittent Fasting, its benefits, tips to get started and the like. In this section, you will learn about a couple of reasons why Intermittent Fasting is a good idea while traveling.

Efficiency

Let us assume that your flight lands in Frankfurt from New York, but you need to catch a bus, which will take nine hours to meet your pals in Berlin. You need to collect your luggage from the baggage claim, go through the border security, get your bearings, take a cab to the bus station and eat something along the way. Oh wait, you don't have to worry about the last item on your list since you are fasting. It helps you focus on your travel. If you want to reach your destination without any unnecessary delays, then Intermittent Fasting will come in handy.

Save money

If you fast for at least 14 to 16 hours in a day, it means that you can deduct the expenses for at least one meal. If you do this whenever you are traveling, you can save quite a bit. Not just a meal, but you can even reduce your snacking expenses. On an average, you can save anywhere between $30 and $50 per day. So, if you are traveling for a week, you can save close to $300 on your food expenses.

Energy

If you have a sensitive stomach or are used to following a specific diet when you are home, then trying out new foods can upset your stomach. When you fast, you tend to not only save energy but will feel more alert as well. All this energy that you save, you can use while traveling for sightseeing or any other activities.

Control

Things tend to happen - flights or buses can be late, plans can change and you might not speak the local language. You cannot control all these things, but the one thing that you can control is the way you treat your body. Intermittent Fasting will give you a sense of control that you might not otherwise find in a foreign land. Even if you are a frequent traveler, the local culture, language and people can seem quite overwhelming and tiring. If you are used to Intermittent Fasting, then it will give you a sense of routine and normalcy. If you want to hold onto this sense of control, then you simply need to stick to your dieting protocols even when you travel.

Time

Think about all the time that you spend when you need to get food and eat food. In fact, at times, a major portion of your traveling time goes on eating. There is nothing wrong with this. It certainly is exciting trying new things, but the purpose of traveling isn't merely eating. While following the protocols of this diet, you will realize that you have more time to do other activities. All the time that you spend eating is now freed up and you can do whatever you want. Also, if you are in a rush while getting from one place to the next, then at least you don't have to worry about eating.

Cleanse

Intermittent Fasting gives your body an opportunity to cleanse itself. Your body needs a break from all the traveling and the work that you do. Intermittent Fasting is a method of self-cleanse and it is quite simple. When you don't constantly keep pumping food into your system, your system can start cleaning itself.

Chapter Thirteen:

Weight Loss on a Budget

I ntermittent Fasting sounds like a proper diet, doesn't it? It is a proper diet without the unnecessary frills that come along with a conventional diet. Well, there is more good news for you. You can lose weight while on a strict budget. So, you can improve your health and achieve your weight loss goals while you stick to a budget. This does sound good, doesn't it? It sounds even better in a world that is overrun with different expensive fad diets that will burn a hole in your pocket. In this section, you will learn about certain tips that you can follow to shed those excess pounds while on a budget.

Water, water, and more water

It is quite important that your body is always thoroughly hydrated. Water not only hydrates your body, clears your skin, flushes out the toxins, but it also makes you feel fuller for longer. You must drink at least eight glasses of water per day. Regardless of the method of Intermittent Fasting you want to follow, you must drink plenty of water. Whenever you feel a hunger pang strike you, calm yourself down and drink a glass of water. You must always carry a water bottle with you. You can add a sprig of mint leaves and a couple of slices of lemon to the water to spruce it up.

Eat slowly

You need to learn to eat slowly. Never be in a rush to stuff yourself and instead concentrate on what you are eating. When you eat slowly, the urge to binge fades away. You need to chew your food thoroughly before you swallow it. If you eat slowly, it helps improve the process of digestion and absorption of food. Learn to savor the flavors of the food, the textures and the smells. Try to be mindful of what you are eating, and you can slow yourself down.

Eat healthily

Intermittent Fasting primarily concentrates on when you eat and not what you eat. It doesn't mean that you are free to eat anything that you please. If you want to lead a healthy life and achieve your weight loss objectives, then you need to eat healthy and wholesome meals. The meals that you eat must provide your body the nourishment it needs.

Cook at home

Try to cook at home as often as you can. If you want to save some money on your food bills, then avoid buying prepacked meals. It might seem quite easy to order a salad, but it will be quite expensive in the long run. You don't need any fancy ingredients while following Intermittent Fasting, so you don't have to buy a lot of groceries. You can cook simple meals and home and ensure that you eat at home. Instead of ordering a $10 salad, you can buy a big bag of mixed salad greens for $5 and have two meals instead of one!

Ration your portions

You must control the portions you eat. You can do this by weighing out the portions you eat. The meals you consume need to be rich in protein and fiber, while low in carbs. If you eat plenty of fiber, protein and the right amount of dietary fats, then your body will obtain all the necessary nutrients that it needs to stay healthy.

Plan your meals

With Intermittent Fasting, you can select your eating window. When you know this, you can easily plan for your meals in advance. If you know that you will be fasting all day long, then make sure that there is a tasty meal waiting for you at home. By doing this, you will effectively reduce the urge to eat out.

Grocery shopping

Grocery shopping might seem like a chore, but it is quite important. Before you decide to head out, you need to make a list of all the groceries that you need. You don't need any junk food or unhealthy foods stored at home if you are trying to eat healthily. So, the first thing that you need to do is clear your pantry off all the food items that aren't healthy. Also, you must never shop when you are hungry.

You must not only prepare a food list, but you need to make sure that you stick to it while shopping. It is quite easy to cook if you have all the necessary ingredients readily available. Shop for your groceries once a week and if you plan your meals in advance, you will know the groceries you need to buy.

Meal prep

You must make it a habit of doing the basic meal prep over the weekends. It helps you prepare for the week that lies ahead. Meal prep is quite simple, and it can something as basic as cutting or chopping up vegetables. You can make a couple of simple curry pastes or stews and freeze them. You can even partially cook meats and freeze them. You can pretty much freeze anything that you want. For instance, you can make a Thai curry paste and freeze it. So, on a weekday, you merely need to add some protein and vegetables to the curry paste and voila, your meal is ready.

One of the best things that you can cook in batches and freeze is broth! You can use the broth to make soups, stews, and curries.

Eat fruit for dessert

If you have a sweet tooth, it might feel challenging to give up on desserts. So, to satiate your sweet cravings, you can have fruit for dessert. A cup of strawberries with a tablespoon of unsweetened whipped cream is a tasty dessert. Have berries or any other fruit that you want. Fruit is good for your body and are full of nutrients. However, you must be mindful of the hidden calories they consist of. You must not have three mangoes just because it is a fruit. Eat healthily! For instance, frozen bananas with some peanut butter, or apple wedges with peanut butter make for a tasty sweet treat. There are plenty of healthy alternatives for desserts and try them out.

Food budget

You must set a weekly or a monthly food budget for yourself. It isn't about merely setting a budget, but you also need to make sure that you stick to the budget. When you are planning your food budget, you need to make sufficient allocations for grocery shopping. It helps you keep a track of your expenses. You can always download a mobile application to track your spending.

Eat the healthy stuff first

Whenever you break your fast, you might be overcome by the urge to eat a lot of food. Your body might start craving for carbs and sugar. So, you need to make sure that you eat all the healthy stuff before you even think about eating anything unhealthy. If you want a scoop of ice cream or a bar of chocolate, you must tell yourself that you can eat that stuff after you eat all the necessary protein and fiber. Once your tummy is full, then the urge to eat will also reduce. If you do this, you will not feel like you are denying yourself anything.

Brush your teeth after eating

It is a healthy habit to brush your teeth before you go to sleep at night. Ensure that you brush your teeth after dinner. In a way, it is a signal to your body that you have finished with the meals for any given day. It certainly helps on a psychological level. Not only will you have stronger and cleaner teeth, but it also reduces the urge to want to eat.

Don't leave the house hungry

You must never leave the house hungry. How often do you purchase a cup of coffee on your way to work? Coffee will certainly wake you up in the morning, but how much do you spend on your morning fix-me up? If you are used to buying coffee daily, then you will spend about $5 in one go. That's about $150 a month and $1800 a year! That's a lot of money that you can use for something else. Instead, why don't you brew your coffee at home and take it along with you? That's not only simple but is quite inexpensive as well.

Also, you must never leave the house hungry. If your fasting period ends and you want to head out for a meal, make sure that you snack on something healthy before heading out.

Make your snacks

You don't have to buy diet snacks anymore. You can make your own 100-calorie snacks at home and carry them with you. It is quite easy to make your own snacks at home. For instance, it doesn't take more than ten minutes to whip up a batch of kale chips or popcorn. You can store them in small containers and eat whenever you are hungry.

Track what you eat

You can maintain a food journal or use one of the food tracking apps to keep tabs on what you eat. The key is to make a list of everything that you eat. It will help you to eat healthily and cut down on any mindless snacking. When you start tracking what you eat, you will automatically become conscious of the things you are feeding your body.

Exercise

You don't need an expensive gym membership to exercise. There are plenty of different ways in which you can exercise without heading to the gym. You can go for a run, jog or even do yoga at home.

We all have incredibly hectic schedules and lead busy lives and at such a time, it might be difficult to follow a diet. Well, you no longer have to worry about this. The tips explained in this chapter will help you follow the protocols of Intermittent Fasting without burning a hole in your pocket.

Chapter Fourteen:
Get Lean while Eating Out

Why is Intermittent Fasting so effective? This diet is quite filling. When you skip breakfast and eat at noon, you are giving yourself the necessary room to eat later. Most of us tend to eat a lot of food at night and that's due to a primitive urge present within us. Once you get used to fasting, you will feel quite focused during the morning and will be able to appreciate the food that you eat later. You can do all this while making sure that you are maintaining a calorie deficit.

Another reason for the popularity of this diet is that it is quite simple. In this busy world that we live in, most of us don't have the time to eat five to six perfectly balanced small meals. It just isn't possible. So, the idea of eating two big and filling meals per day fits in with the hectic schedule of our lives. It also offers a certain degree of flexibility that is necessary.

Intermittent Fasting is designed in such a way that it supports your calorie and macronutrient requirements. It means that by following this dieting protocol, it is quite difficult to exceed your calorie intake. The meal plan that you need to follow ensures that you can consume a lot of protein and fiber that makes you feel full and helps you build lean muscle. Because of all this, it is quite easy to meet your weight loss and fitness goals.

In this section, you will learn about a couple of different strategies that you can follow while eating out.

Strategy 1: Nutrition plan

The first thing that you need to do is track your nutritional intake while at home and you must be aware of the number of calories that you consume, the size of the portions and the composition of your meals. For instance, if you consume 1800 calories in three meals, your dinner can make up for 700 calories, lunch for 400 calories and the rest for another meal. It means that you can have about 70g of protein for lunch and dinner and about 40g in another meal.

Strategy 2: Stick to the Same Foods

Once you establish your calculated nutrition plan, it is all about sticking to it as much as you can while eating out. Ideally, you must try to stick to similar foods to those that you eat while at home. For instance, if you are used to a meal of meats and vegetables, then order something similar when you go out for a meal. If you go out for a meal, stick to the protein and fibers you eat at home and skip any carb and sugar-rich foods.

Strategy 3: Increase Protein

If you aren't sure what to eat and cannot decide, a simple thing that you can do is to increase the portion of the protein you order. You can double up the protein and it will help make you feel full. It isn't just about picking a protein, but you need to pick the protein wisely. It doesn't make any sense if you binge on fried chicken or ribs slathered in barbeque sauce. Avoid all the high-calorie options on the menu. Instead, you must opt for leaner meats like lamb, steak, chicken or fish.

Strategy 4: Carbs

You need to be careful about the amount of carbs you consume. If the dish you ordered has more carbohydrates than you are used to consuming, then simply skip the carbs. You need to avoid carbs as much as possible if you want to speed up the process of weight loss. Carbs will fill you up for a while and then you will feel hungry again. Instead, fill up on the foods that are good for you. If there is a breadbasket on the table, please resist the urge of reaching for it.

Strategy 5: Post Meal Hunger

If you want to have a dessert or still have the urge to eat more, even though you are aware that it will exceed your ideal calorie intake, then you need to know that this feeling of hunger will subside soon. A simple trick is to have a cup of tea after a meal and it will make you feel full. You can also go for a walk after eating and you will feel full. It takes about 20 minutes for your brain to signal to you that you are full so don't keep stuffing yourself with food.

If you follow these simple steps, you can stick to your diet even when you go out for a meal.

Chapter Fifteen:

How to set up a Plan (i.e. 8-Week Meal Plan)

L et's get started with making a plan for your Intermittent Fasting. A good plan will be your guide on what you should do and how you should maintain your diet. There are a few steps to creating the perfect plan for your body. First choose the fasting method that you think you can work with. Decide the duration and frequency that you want to fast for.

Think of your eating habits in general and choose from the type of Intermittent Fasting that will suit you. If one type doesn't suit you, just change and try another. There is no harm in trying out what works best for you in the long run. You need to notice your usual eating habits and decide which type of eating personality you have. Generally, there are three eating personalities amongst people; Type A, Type B and Type C. Use the following information to find out which type applies to you.

- Type A: Consider yourself lucky if you have Type A eating personality. This type of eating makes fasting easy for you. You will find Intermittent Fasting surprisingly simple for you to follow and stick to. Normally if you unintentionally don't eat for long period of time, this is your personality type. It is not the same as intentionally starving yourself so keep that in mind. You are usually the type who gets busy with other things and tends to forget meals until hunger really strikes. Type A people generally don't tend to try any random diets and fasting might be a first for them. You also don't feel anxious and compulsive about food. If all of this is true for you, you now know your eating personality type.

- Type B: People with this eating personality like to make sure that they eat all their meals on time. It is usually embedded in your mind that you need to eat every single proper meal and get anxious if you miss any. You also are not comfortable about going on any diets and don't do well when you try a diet. Type B personalities always try to make up for skipped meals even when they aren't hungry.

- Type C: Intermittent Fasting is usually the most difficult for people with the tendencies of Type C. However, this is the type that tends to try out diets the most and usually fails. You might be binge eating and have cravings all the time. Type C also don't like missing any meals and eat to make up for any skipped meals. You get anxious and think too much about when and what you will eat. This type of eating personality generally tends to overeat and has weight issues over time.

However, Intermittent Fasting will work for you no matter which type of eating personality you have. It just helps you to define what your eating habits are and how you should try this type of fast. For Type C eating personality, it is recommended to go slow and try your best to stick to the plan but without stressing out about any missed days. The other two types can usually start out with at least 2 days of fasting a week even from their first day. No matter what your type is, just make a plan that you are comfortable with and motivate yourself to stick to it in order to reach your end goal.

A Type A eating personality makes it easy for you to start any fasting diet plan right away. You will see that it is not too different from your usual habits but don't overdo it. Set memos that will remind you to eat on time. Starving yourself for too long will do more harm than good. Try two days of 20-hour fasts on the first week and add another day to this the second week.

Type B eating personality people should go a little slower than Type A. Slowly build up the pace of your fasting without stressing too much about it. Getting anxious about food is not healthy. You can start with 18-20 hour fasts on the first week and do the same the second week but try to add a couple of hours to it.

Type C eating personality people need to be more cautious about their fasting. You need to take it at a slow pace so that it does not overwhelm you but also make sure that you don't give up too soon. You have to build a plan that you know you can stick to. Don't set unrealistic goals or expect too much from yourself. If you try to fast the same as Type A and B people you will actually trigger binge eating quite soon into your plan. Instead take it a day at a time. On days that you feel you can't, just let it go but adjust it the next day. Set goals for every week. For the first week try an 18-hour fast for one day. Enjoy your normal eating on the other days but be a little conscious about trying to compensate for the day you fasted or will fast again. Don't eat too much just when you break your fast. The next week make it an 18-hour fast on 2 days of the week with at least two days of rest in between these. Fasting for too long will make you sick. Try to be determined for the course of the fasting that you decide on.

Decide on the day that you want to start your fasting. Once you decide, don't budge on it and begin on that very day. Keep some drinks that are non-calorific around. Remember to stay hydrated even if you aren't eating. Water is essential for your body. Keep a timer on your phone to mark the end of your fast. This way you can expect a notification for when you can eat again.

If you are a Type A personality for eating, then begin with an 18-hour fast in your first week and then a 24-hour fast.

If you want to try at least 15-hour fasts on a daily basis, keep these on alternate days for your first week of fasting. If you are a Type B personality for eating then try a 16-hour fast after dinner on your first week. Let it last until lunchtime the next day. Then try to increase a couple of hours and try again after a few days. The next week you can try to make it a 24-hour fast.

For Type C personalities, try a 16-hour fast from evening until 10 a.m. the next day on your first week. Then try again the next week and try to do this twice in a week. Let it build up as you go from there.

Take some notes during your fasting for the first two times. Write down how you felt both physically and mentally.

If you feel sick or nauseous at any point, we recommend consulting the doctor.

Let's take a look at a sample plan to get started. This particular plan is more suitable for anyone who just wants to get a head start on Intermittent Fasting and wants to continue it as a part of their lifestyle.

Week One

Let's assume you start fasting on a Sunday. Begin after dinner around 7 p.m. Then keep fasting until 1 p.m. on Monday. Don't fast on this Tuesday and eat like you normally would. Keep your Wednesday fast free as well. On Thursday start fasting after lunch around 1 p.m. and fast until lunchtime on Friday. Do not fast on this next Saturday and Sunday. If the first day was too hard for you, just keep it as one day of fasting for the first week.

When you begin, you need to remember to pace your body. Don't ever fast for two days in a row. Keep a gap of at least two days between each fast. If the hours were too long for your first few days, just reduce a couple and adjust according to your capacity. You can build it up over the next few weeks. The goal is to focus long-term benefits and not short-term failures.

Week Two'

For this second week, keep your first week experience in mind. Decide on the hours that you think will suit you this week and try to increase it even if for one hour. Make the fasting fit around your lifestyle. Choose the days that would suit you and your work and commitments. We are just giving you a sample that you can work with.

This Sunday start fasting after dinner around 9 p.m. and fast until 7 p.m. on Monday. Try to implement a 24-hour fast for this second week if you feel up to it. Don't fast for Tuesday or Wednesday. Eat lunch and start fasting around 1 p.m. on Thursday and break the fast at 1 p.m. on Friday. Don't fast any more for your second week. Don't overeat after your fast is over. This means that you fast for 2 days on your second week.

Week Three

If week two went as planned, you can adjust and increase your times for week three. Start fasting after dinner on Sunday around 9 p.m. Then break the fast around 1 p.m. on Monday. Eat healthy meals for this next two days. On Wednesday, start fasting after lunch around 3 p.m. and break it on Thursday for breakfast around 10am. The next fast should be for half a day from Friday night after dinner at 9 p.m. to 9 a.m. the next day. This just gives you a few extra hours this week to fast.

Week Four

This week try fasting for a few days in shorter intervals. Begin your fast at 8 p.m. on Sunday night and break it by 1 p.m. on Monday. Then fast from 8 p.m. on Tuesday until 1 p.m. on Wednesday and fast again from Thursday from 8 p.m. to Friday until 1 p.m. These will help give you another kind of pace.

Week Five

This week you can start trying to fast every day for 16-18 hours other than the weekend. Eat like you normally do until Sunday dinner and fast from 8 p.m. until 12 p.m. on Monday. Until Friday you have to fast every day and you are allowed to eat only from 12 p.m. to 7 p.m. each day. The 18 hours in between each day's intervals will be for fasting. On Saturday and Sunday give yourself a break. If you couldn't do every single day, take a break in between and don't feel guilty.

Week Six

See how week five went for you. Were you able to try the fast on all the weekdays? You actually get to eat both lunch and dinner for this. If it did not work and you took some days off, try the same routine as week five for week six. Give your body and mind another chance to tough it out.

Week Seven

I'm sure you have the hang of it by now. You can see how it gets easier over time. Try fasting on every alternate day this week. Don't let your body get used to one particular routine. This way you won't have to lead a very strict schedule. Fast from Sunday 7 p.m. to Monday 12 p.m. don't fast until Tuesday 8 p.m. again and repeat these steps for every other day. This week will be much easier. Try to get some exercise in when you are not fasting. Exercising on fasting days will be too taxing for your body.

Week Eight

This is the last week for your set plan. If you have been eating healthy and following the fasting plan, you have already seen changes. It should now be much easier to fast for hours at a time. Week Seven was a break so fast a little extra for this final week.

Start fasting on Sunday at 8 p.m. and eat at 1 p.m. on Monday. Then fast from Monday 8 p.m. until 5 p.m. on Tuesday. Start a fast at 1 p.m. after lunch on Wednesday and break it at dinner on that day. Don't fast on Thursday and then fast from Thursday 8 p.m. until 5 p.m. on Friday. Take a break from fasting now.

You will notice how each week, it gets much easier to follow a plan. The plan helps you mark out what times you can eat and when you can't. It helps you avoid binge eating and reaching for snacks without considering the time. You can eat normally when you are not fasting. But remember not to overeat the meal right after you break your fast. Give your body time to adjust. Also, don't think that you can reward yourself too much after a fast. You should still try to watch what you are eating during your eating intervals. If you load up on too many carbs during your meals, your weight will not show much change. These first few weeks are important to create a healthier lifestyle for yourself. Use the schedule to discipline yourself. There is still a lot of room for adjustment as you go from week one to eight. After you finish week eight, you can decide what type of Intermittent Fasting works best for you. Try to make a plan every month on how you want to keep implementing fasting in your habits. Mark down the events and occasions that you want to enjoy with your family or friends eating good food. It's a good idea to fast on the day after such events. Hydrate yourself with water and herbal teas during your fast. Avoid overeating whether you are at home or away from home. Overeating encourages a type of compulsive eating that you need to learn to grow out of. The Intermittent Fasting helps curb such habits when you know you aren't supposed to touch food during specific hours. So, don't undo all your hard work in a moment of weakness. Learn from the experience.

After your eight weeks, you will see how your body looks and feels differently. Healthier eating always has a good impact on the body. You have probably been drinking a lot of water as well and this can make the appearance of your skin much better. If your want proof of the health benefits, why not go to a doctor before and after these eight weeks of planned Intermittent Fasting? They can help to show you the difference it has made. Your energy levels will be much higher than when you used to overeat every single day. Don't live to eat, eat to live but you can still enjoy the foods you love. Let your food and habits improve the state of your mind and body. Fasting allows your body time to actually use up the reserved energy and food you have consumed. It also makes you feel more conscious of everything you do and you will see improvements all around.

Give it a chance and follow the fasting timings that are given above. It allows you to slowly make fasting a part of your life without burdening you like other diets. You don't have to throw out your favorite chocolates and stop eating your cookies. You just have to learn to eat as much as your body actually needs and not too often.

Chapter Sixteen:
Keeping Up the Motivation

Now that you know all about Intermittent Fasting, you've probably tried it for at least a week or two. But are you frustrated because you aren't seeing any visible results? Do you feel like you haven't lost any weight? Or even worse, do you feel like you have gained some?

Intermittent Fasting is not like other fad diets that assure you of weight loss in a few days. You won't see quick results that will make you want to keep doing it until you reach your goal weight. It is a diet that needs patience and will show you results in time according to your body. You need to let your body lose weight in a healthy way and not by trying to rush it. Even if you feel negative because of the rise in the weight scale, there are a few normal reasons for it. Give it time and you will see the opposite happen in a few weeks. Consistency is key to anything. If you don't persist in going through the diet properly, you can't expect to see results.

Let's look at how you can keep yourself motivated in the long run. Start focusing on what's going right in your life and not what's wrong with it. This diet is just a part of it. Just starting with the diet means that you are taking a step in the right direction. Focus on going through all your regular activities and work that needs to be done. Get those completed and stay patient with your fasting diet. In fact, fasting actually gives you more time to focus on other things. The end of the fast has a different effect on your body and you will feel it.

Intermittent Fasting also helps to build your self-discipline and self-control. Every day that you fast allows you to see how far you can go and control your usual instincts. Reaching out for snacks or any food is quite instinctive and that is why people gain a lot of weight. You, on the other hand, know what's right and are trying to keep your body healthy. Even if you have cravings in the middle of the day, you are still suppressing them and make it through to the night. You need to remind yourself and appreciate that you are doing your best every day. Going through each day until the end of your diet plan is what will help you see weight loss and a better body.

When you can't depend on yourself or feel like you aren't sure of the diet, look for inspiration in others. There are lots of other people who have tried the Intermittent Fasting diet and have watched it work for them. There are books, articles, YouTube videos, etc. that are proof of their successful results. People who struggle with weight loss often share their journey. When you see their stories, you will realize that instant gratification is not the way to a fit body. You need to have control over your diet and habits. That is the only way you can achieve the goal you set for yourself.

There are many benefits that you can reap from Intermittent Fasting other than weight loss. It has been shown to help detoxify your body, regulate blood sugar levels, improve brain health, etc. It is not just about losing weight. You need to lose some unwanted fat and gain muscle. This might be the same weight on the scale but it will produce a different and better body shape. The same number will still show changes in the measurements of your body. You will feel and look a lot different over time and this is the healthy change you need to aim for. So, don't lose hope too soon.

You have to remember that weight loss is a journey that will give you bad days and good days. You need to stay strong and determined if you want the Intermittent Fasting to work for you. Try to enjoy the process and you will reap the fruits of your hard work.

Chapter Seventeen:
How to Keep the Weight Stable

I f your main goal with Intermittent Fasting is to lose weight, you need to keep some things in mind. Weight loss is a process and after that you need to still balance your habits to keep in good shape. If you follow the diet right and work with it, you will definitely see the weight loss in a few weeks. However, your goal should be long-term fitness and health benefits. If you think you can get back to your old habits right after the diet is over, you're wrong. You can eat what you want during and after the diet but it is important to keep your self-control. You learn how to control unhealthy eating with the help of Intermittent Fasting. This is something your mind and body will remember even after your 8-week plan is over. So, utilize your new habits and exercise the self-control needed to stay in good health.

Don't make things too hard on yourself. Unlike other diets, this diet allows you to be flexible. If you have a dinner planned with your friends on a fasting day, just go for it. You can still make up for it later. The point is not to eat too much unnecessarily every single day. Fasting after a night out will help you detoxify if you make it a habit once in a while. If you want to make a plan for yourself, keep any family events in mind and mark other days for fasting. This way you won't miss out on what you want and if you do, you will just be more likely to give up the diet altogether at some point. Be kind to yourself, changes take time.

Don't be extreme in trying to lose weight. Learn to love your body and try to include healthy habits to show it the care it deserves. Stay away from any fad diets that tell you to stop eating for a week or to just drink juices. These will never help you in the long term and can actually harm your body. Eat the food you love from time to time so that you can avoid binge eating. Forbidden things are always a temptation. Instead of overdoing it, just eat a little once in a while so that you don't think about it or have any unhealthy cravings on your fasting days.

Be realistic about your diet and expectations. Also try to add some sort of physical exercise every single day. Even if you just go for a walk, it counts for something. It is not necessary to hit the gym every day like a fanatic but if you like it, then it will definitely speed up the process. Exercise keeps your system running well and your body fit. If you like waking up early then why not try a run around the park. One of the best ways to keep yourself motivated is to do this with a friend. You won't get bored and you can depend on someone to check up on you once in a while. Make it as easy for yourself as possible. You don't have to exert yourself beyond your limits. Don't believe anyone who tries to tell you that you have to hit the gym twice a day to get the body you want. In fact, too much exercise can actually harm you. Just think of it as a simple activity you can inculcate in your routine a few times a week to keep your blood pumping.

Chapter Eighteen:
Busting Intermittent Fasting Myths

I ntermittent Fasting has immense benefits. Although the concept of going without food for longer periods may seem dreadful to many, fasting has time and again proved to be greatly beneficial for human health. Not eating for longer periods is not only therapeutic for the body, but also boosts a person's immune system, enhances person's insulin sensitivity, recycles old damaged cells, improved DNA repair and offers protection against many other disease. But the most talked about benefits of Intermittent Fasting is weight loss.

The increasing popularity of Intermittent Fasting has also given rise to some myths. Below, we are going to bust some of the most common myths about snacking, fasting and meal frequency.

Skipping breakfast makes you fat

For years, we have been fed this belief that "Breakfast is the most important meal of the day." How many of us question the authenticity of this question? I bet not many. Most people believe that skipping breakfast can result in cravings, hunger and even weight gain in some cases. While a lot of observational researchers have found statistical links between obesity and skipping breakfast, it could be that the quintessential breakfast skipper may not be a health-conscious person overall. A study was published in 2014 that compared people who ate breakfast versus people who skipped breakfast. The 16-week study concluded that there was no significant weight loss difference between the two groups. That said, there have been certain studies, which show that teenagers and children might benefit from eating breakfast by performing better at school. Eating breakfast could be beneficial for some people while for others it might not be as beneficial.

Increase in the frequency of meals helps to boost your metabolism

A lot of nutritionists believe that eating small meals throughout the day can help to accelerate your metabolism. It's certainly true that the human body can expand some amount of energy by assimilating and digesting the nutrients in a meal. This phenomenon is known as the thermic food effect (TEF) which adds up to 30% calories for protein, between 0-3 % for fats and 5-10% for carbohydrates. Overall, the impact of the thermic food is about 10% of a person's total calorie intake. Here, what actually matters is not the amount of meals you consume, but the actual calories that were consumed.

When you eat seven 400-calorie meals in a day, it has a similar effect as eating three 700-calorie meals a day. If you measure the thermic effect here, of 10%, it amounts to 210 calorie in both cases. This fact has also been supported by several feeding studies conducted on humans which show that the increase of decrease in meal frequency is not associated or has no impact on the total calories burned.

Eating frequently prevents you from over eating and reduces hunger

Some of us believe that frequent snacking can help reduce cravings or prevent hunger. When you look at some of the studies conducted on this belief, there has been an interesting mix of evidence. While some studies have shown that an increased frequency in meals results in reduced hunger, others show an increased level of hunger. A particular study that compared 6 high protein meals and 3 high protein meals, it was found that the 3 high-protein meals were more effective in reducing hunger in the participants. However, such an impact could totally vary from person to person. If you feel that snacking helps you stay away from cravings or reduces the chances of you binging, then go for it no matter what the studies say.

There has been no scientific evidence that snacking often or consuming frequent meals can guarantee reduction in your hunger pangs. You can choose what works for you.

Smaller meals can help you lose weight

There has been no evidence that smaller meals boost your metabolism. They also do not contribute toward reducing your hunger pangs. If you consider the fact that consuming frequent meals has no impact on the energy balance equation, then technically it won't have any impact on weight loss either. This fact was also supported scientifically. Several studies that were conducted on his topic showed that meal frequency has no impact on weight loss.

For instance, a research that was conducted involving 16 obese males and females showed that none of the participants experienced any difference in fat loss, weight or appetite when comparing 6 or 3 meals each day.
That said - you might find that eating smaller meals more frequently can make it easier for you to control your cravings, then this could be effective for you. It's also possible that if you have digestion issues, then you can benefit from breaking down your meals in smaller meals. In general, I find

it difficult to eat so often which makes it harder for me to control my diet. But it may work for some people.

Your brain requires a constant supply of glucose

We have always believed that eating carbs every few hours is the only way to keep our brains functioning well. This belief could be rooted in the fact that our brains use only glucose as a source of fuel. However, what we don't discuss is that our body is capable of easily producing glucose it requires via a process called gluconeogenesis. Now, this is not required in all cases as your body is already used to storing glycogen in the liver. These glycogen stores can be used to provide enough energy for the brain for hours.

The same goes for long-term fasting. Even when you fast for longer hours, consume a low-carbohydrate diet or starve, your body can produce ketones from dietary fats. Ketone bodies are known for offering energy for most part of the brain while being able to reduce its glucose requirement completely. So, when a person fasts, his or her brain is easily able to sustain by using the ketones as well as the glucose that is produced from fats and proteins.

If you look at it form an evolutionary perspective, the belief that humans wouldn't be able to survive without a consistent supply of carbohydrates is completely senseless. If this fact were true, then the human species would have become extinct a long time ago.

That said - some people might feel hypoglycemic if they go longer periods without eating anything. If you have had the same experience, then you should consume more and more meals throughout the day. But before you make any dietary changes, do consult your doctor and ask for his suggestions regarding this dietary approach.

Snacking and eating frequently is good for health

It is unnatural for the body to stay in a constantly fed state. Back in the day when humans were still evolving, they had to experience food scarcity quite frequently. Scientifically, there has been some evidence suggesting that short-term fasting can trigger a cellular repair phase called autophagy. What is autophagy? It's a process where the human cells make use of dysfunctional and old proteins for energy.

Autophagy is known to help protect humans from developing diseases such as Alzheimer's disease, cancer or even help reduce signs of aging. The fact is that fasting has time and again proved to be beneficial for our metabolic health. Some studies have shown that eating often and snacking can in fact have a negative impact on human health. For instance, one particular research has shown that frequent meals along with a high calorie intake can result in increased liver fat, implying that snacking often can increase the risk of developing fatty liver disease. Some observations studies have also proved that people who snack often or eat frequent meals are at a higher risk of developing colorectal cancer.

Fasting puts your body in starvation mode

This is one of the most common myths against Intermittent Fasting. A lot of people seem to believe that Intermittent Fasting can put you in starvation mode. As per a lot of claims, when you don't eat, your body thinks that it is starving, so it starts shutting down the metabolism which further hinders you from burning fat. Long-term weight loss can certainly cause a reduction in the amount of calories you burn and put you in starvation mode. This impact can cause less calories to be burned each day.

However, this effect takes place with weight loss regardless of the technique you use. There has been no evidence showing that this only happens when you are fasting or that it doesn't happen with other weight loss methods. So, it's a bit unfair to single out Intermittent Fasting. In fact, there has been some evidence that shows short-term fasts can result in an increase in metabolic rate. This generally happens due to a spike in norepinephrine content in the blood which causes break down of body fat while stimulating a person's metabolism.

Several studies have shown that when you fast up to 48 hours, your metabolism gets a boost of 3.6-14%. But when someone fasts longer than that then the chances are the impact can reverse, causing the metabolism to go down as compared to the baseline.

Your body is capable of using only a certain amount of protein for each meal

This is another topic that has been debated over the years. There are some people who claim that humans are only capable of digesting 30 grams of protein per meal. They also suggest that eating every 2 or 3 hours can help maximize muscle gain. That said - this theory is not supported by science. Studies do not have any evidence that there is a difference in muscle mass of a person if she or he consumes protein in smaller doses. Time and again, it has been proved that it's the total amount of protein consumed by us matters and not the amount of meals it's spread over.

Fasting can make you lose muscle

The common belief is that fasting can make our bodies lose muscle and start using it as fuel. While there's some truth to this phenomenon when people diet in general, there has been no specific evidence that it occurs more with fasting as compared to other weight loss methods. In fact, there have been certain studies which suggest that fasting can actually be largely beneficial for maintaining muscle mass.

In a particular study, intermittent calorie restriction resulted in the same amount of weight loss like calorie restriction. However, there was less reduction in muscle mass. Another study was conducted involving participants who consumed the same amount of calories as before only exception of one big meal in the evening. These participants lost a lot of body fat while having a modest amount of increase in their muscle mass. They also experienced a lot of other health benefits due to fasting.

Intermittent Fasting is also extremely popular particularly among bodybuilders who found it to be effective in maintaining high amounts of muscle while having a low body fat percentage.

Fasting is bad for our health

A lot of people assume that fasting does more harm to the body than good. But this couldn't be further from the truth. Several studies have shown that Intermittent Fasting as well as intermittent calorie restriction can offer impressive health benefits. For instance, Intermittent Fasting can cause the expression of genes linked with longevity to undergo a change and has proven to prolong lifespan in animals. Fasting also offers a lot of benefits for our metabolic health, which includes reduction in oxidative stress, insulin sensitivity, and reduction in the possibility of heart disease.

It has also been found that fasting can actually benefit our brain health by boosting a hormone known as rain-derived neurotropic factor (BDNF). This can be used to protect us against depression as well as other brain-related issues.

Intermittent Fasting makes us overeat

There are some claims that suggest that Intermittent Fasting, instead of causing weight loss, makes us lose weight, as fasting tends to make you overeat during the eating periods. This is true, but only in part. In short, people only end up compensating for the calories that are lost during fasting by consuming more food during the eating window.

That said, this compensation isn't absolute. One particular study has shown that participants who fasted for an entire day ended up consuming an additional 500 calories the next day. These participants expended 2400 calories approximately during the fasting period and ended up overeating by 500 calories the day after. If you so the math, the total reduction in their calorie intake was about 1900 calories and this is a huge deficit considering it's only for 2 days.

The truth is that Intermittent Fasting is one of the most effective tools to lose weight. Stating that starvation can make you overeat and gain weight is completely untrue.

Conclusion

I want to thank you once again for purchasing this book and I hope you enjoyed it.

Intermittent Fasting is a great diet, isn't it? Fasting for extended periods can help achieve your weight loss goals while improving your overall health. Intermittent Fasting is a flexible diet and you can customize it according to your lifestyle needs and convenience.

There are multiple benefits this diet offers. Select a fasting protocol that you can easily incorporate into your daily schedule. If you can add a little exercise to your schedule, you can even build lean muscle! So, all that you need to do now is get started as soon as possible!

CPSIA information can be obtained
at www.ICGtesting.com
Printed in the USA
BVHW042023210421
605394BV00011BA/1963